CONTENTS

INTRODUCTION

Did you know that inflammation can take a significant toll on your body?

Inflammation is a very serious problem, but most people don't even know what it is. When it comes to the body, inflammation refers to a process that occurs when your white blood cells are activated to protect your body from infections, viruses, and bacteria. This means inflammation isn't always a bad thing. It's a natural response that can keep your body protected. However, when things get out of control and the inflammation in your body doesn't go away (which it naturally should when the threat is gone), that's when problems may arise.

Chronic inflammation is one of the most common factors associated with diseases like diabetes, arthritis, bowel diseases, heart disease, and even cancer. It can also cause you to always feel "off" even if you don't have any diagnosed illnesses. If you suffer from such diseases, if you are at risk for them, or if you feel like you need to make a change to prevent inflammation, you are in the right place. This book will introduce you to the anti-inflammatory diet—a special diet that involves choosing anti-inflammatory foods to help your body heal and become healthier.

Your diet plays an important role in reducing the inflammation occurring in your body. If you keep consuming foods that promote inflammation, you will eventually feel the effects of these foods—you might already be feeling them now. The good news is, it's not too late to start making healthier food choices.

Since food has a dramatic effect on inflammation in the body, you need to focus on consuming anti-inflammatory foods. These types of foods can either reduce or even prevent chronic inflammation. If you suffer from any type of condition that causes inflammation, you definitely need these foods in your life. While medications and other treatments can help you manage your condition, changing your diet can help make things easier for you by improving your overall quality of life. For instance, if you suffer from rheumatoid arthritis, transitioning to an anti-inflammatory diet can reduce the frequency of your flare-ups. Or it can even help lower the level of pain you feel when your flare-ups strike. This diet can help no matter what condition you have, because it will start making positive changes within your body.

In other words, you will transform your body from the inside. Personally speaking, I strongly believe in the power of this healthy diet. When I was in my early twenties, I didn't really think about the foods I ate. I loved fried foods, I couldn't get enough of sweets, and I frequently overindulged in foods that were considered unhealthy. A decade later, I started feeling the effects, and this made me extremely worried. I always felt like there was something wrong with me, but I couldn't pinpoint what it was. Finally, I had myself checked—and that's when I learned that I was at risk for diabetes and heart disease.

At such a young age, I couldn't believe it! I had a long conversation with my doctor about these conditions and, fortunately, my doctor told me that making certain lifestyle choices can help reduce this risk. I started exercising, I made sure that I got enough sleep each night, and I learned how to manage stress more effectively. But the most significant change I made was transitioning to an anti-inflammatory diet. I also did my own research. I learned everything I could about anti-inflammatory foods, as well as the foods that promote inflammation. Then I consulted with a professional nutritionist and a dietitian. They helped me learn how to make wiser dietary choices, and they also helped me learn the art of meal planning—something you will learn here, too.

For so long, I researched, tried new things, experimented with methods, failed, learned from my failures, and I kept going. Now, I feel renewed and rejuvenated. During my last check-up, my doctor congratulated me as he saw the good changes my new diet and lifestyle had made to my health. I have become healthier than ever before and because of this, I felt inspired to write a book about everything I had learned from the experts and everything I had experienced throughout my ongoing anti-inflammatory journey. I want to help you and other people to discover the wonderful benefits of anti-inflammatory foods and the anti-inflammatory diet.

This diet has so many benefits to offer. By following this diet, you can reduce your risk of developing chronic inflammation and all of the diseases associated with it. When this happens, your body can use inflammation properly to protect against infections, injuries, and toxins, instead of causing more harm to your health. By the end of this book, I promise that you will have a clearer picture of what inflammation really is, how it can harm your body, and how you can protect yourself by choosing the right foods. Since food plays an important role in your health, especially in terms of inflammation, it's time for you to start making changes to your diet.

There is no time like the present to make these changes. The more you eat inflammatory foods, the more you are putting yourself at risk. You don't want to end up like me and the countless others who only discovered the benefits of the anti-inflammatory diet because we started feeling the symptoms of chronic inflammation. And if you are already in such a situation, you need this book even more! So, let's begin your anti-inflammatory journey together. If you're ready for it, turn the page to discover how to improve your health, well-being, and the overall quality of your life...

CHAPTER 1: ALL ABOUT THE ANTI-INFLAMMATORY DIET

Before we dive into the specifics of the anti-inflammatory diet, you must first understand what inflammation is all about. Right now, you might be wondering why this diet is so important or why you need to follow it. The term 'inflammation' typically comes with a negative connotation, but the truth is, inflammation is a natural response or process in the body. Without it, your body cannot protect itself from things that can cause harm. But once inflammation gets out of control, things will start going downhill. In this chapter, you will learn the truth about inflammation, along with an introduction to the anti-inflammatory diet and how to start following it.

The Inner Workings of Your Immune System

Inflammation doesn't just refer to something that grows in size. In the body, inflammation is a healthy response of the immune system to viruses, injuries, and infections. Whenever your body is damaged or becomes infected, the immune system triggers inflammation as part of the process of healing. Inflammation can also be a protective response that involves molecular mediators, immune cells, and blood vessels. In this case, inflammation is meant to eliminate damaged tissues, clear out the primary causes of injuries to the cells, purge dead cells, and initiate the process of tissue repair. As you can see, inflammation is very important. This type of natural and beneficial inflammation is known as acute inflammation. Our body needs acute inflammation, which always dies down when the body goes back to normal.

However, when inflammation in your body sticks around despite the absence of infections or any other threats, this is known as chronic inflammation—the bad type of inflammation that is associated with various health conditions. There are several reasons why chronic inflammation may occur, including:

- The presence of some type of autoimmune disorder such as multiple sclerosis, celiac disease, or type 1 diabetes, for example.
- When your body isn't able to eliminate the agent that causes inflammation, like in the case of food sensitivities.
- When you are experiencing chronic stress.
- When you are constantly exposed to low levels of irritants, like environmental pollutants or toxic chemicals that you aren't aware of.

If you can identify what is causing your chronic inflammation, you can determine how to overcome it. If you think that you are suffering from chronic inflammation, you should speak to your doctor about it. This is what I did when I felt like there was always something wrong with me. When my doctor told me that I was already at risk, it opened my eyes and forced me to reevaluate my lifestyle choices. Making a transition to the anti-inflammatory diet even before you are diagnosed with chronic inflammation or any other type of disease associated with inflammation is your healthiest option. This means that you can avoid chronic inflammation altogether so your body can use inflammation correctly.

The anti-inflammatory diet focuses on fruits, veggies, whole grains, healthy fats, lean protein, herbs, spices, and foods that contain omega-3 fatty acids. It also aims to minimize or eliminate the consumption of excess alcohol, red meat, and processed food products. Although it is called a 'diet,' concentrating on anti-inflammatory foods is more of an eating style. You don't have to follow strict guidelines. Instead, you learn how to consciously make healthier choices when it comes to food.

What Causes Chronic Inflammation?

Now that you know that inflammation is a natural response of the body, you don't have to see it as a negative thing. Instead, you must accept that inflammation occurs and make sure that it only occurs when it's needed. Otherwise, if inflammation keeps occurring within your body or if it never goes away, this would indicate that you already suffer from chronic inflammation.

The 'good' type of inflammation, acute inflammation, is the pain, swelling, warmth, and redness that appears around joints or tissues when you get injured. This happens when your immune system releases white blood cells in response to the injury. These white blood cells surround the site of the injury to keep the whole area protected. Through acute inflammation, injuries and infections can heal faster and more efficiently.

Once your inflammation increases to excessive levels or it doesn't go away even after your infections or injuries are gone, this is considered chronic inflammation. Here, your immune system continuously produces white blood cells and other chemical messengers that keep inflammation around. In other words, your body feels like it's constantly under attack, which is why your immune system is always fighting back. Over time, this type of inflammation will start having adverse effects on your body, and it could even lead to a number of serious health conditions.

This happens because the white blood cells that are constantly being produced by your immune system start attacking your healthy organs and tissues. For instance, if you were overweight or obese, your body would have a lot of visceral fat cells. If you suffered from chronic inflammation, your immune system might consider those cells as a threat so the white blood cells it produces will start attacking those visceral fat cells. In this case, as long as you remain overweight or obese, your body will continue to experience chronic inflammation.

By nature, chronic inflammation can remain for extended periods of time. It causes other diseases to occur and, in turn, these diseases can also cause inflammation to occur. This starts a vicious cycle of damage to your body that you need to put a stop to by making changes to your diet and lifestyle. Aside from illnesses, chronic inflammation can be caused by other factors such as:

- Prolonged (and often unaware) exposure to things that cause irritations or allergic reactions to your body. These can come in the form of chemicals, pollution, or even from the food you eat.
- An autoimmune disorder wherein your immune system attacks healthy tissues in your body.
- An injury or infection that is left untreated. The natural response to such would be acute inflammation, but without treatment, it could lead to chronic inflammation.

- Unhealthy habits like smoking and excessive alcohol consumption, for example.

The challenge with chronic inflammation is that it's different for everyone. Some people might experience severe symptoms that disrupt their lives while others don't notice any symptoms at all. For the latter, this could be more dangerous, because they won't know that they are already suffering from chronic inflammation. Over time, this could lead to the development of a chronic disorder, which would be much more difficult to deal with. Also, there are some cases where chronic inflammation happens without any obvious underlying cause. If you're worried about this (and you should be), some of the most common symptoms to look out for include abdominal pain, fever, fatigue, chest pain, mouth sores, or rashes. If you have been experiencing these symptoms and they don't go away, then you may already be suffering from chronic inflammation.

If you experience acute inflammation, you generally don't have to worry about it since this is your body's natural response. Usually, you can sleep off the symptoms, use a cold compress, or take a pain reliever to ease any discomfort. But if you can handle the pain, it's best to allow your body to heal on its own. Chronic inflammation is more challenging, especially if you don't manifest any symptoms. This is why it's recommended to have regular checkups with your doctor so that they can determine if you are suffering from chronic inflammation even if you don't feel anything. Naturally, if you want to avoid chronic inflammation and all its associated risks, you must get ahead of the game. Start making changes to your lifestyle and your diet. The good news is that you're reading this book, which means you're already on your way to learning how to live a healthier life.

How to Get Rid of Inflammation

Making positive changes to your diet and lifestyle can lower your risk of chronic inflammation. When you constantly eat inflammatory foods, these will start affecting your body negatively. In the same way, if you constantly practice unhealthy habits, chronic inflammation will surely follow close behind. The anti-inflammatory diet is only one aspect of leading a healthier life. Before we go into the specifics of the anti-inflammatory diet, let's discuss the most practical and effective tips to reduce inflammation.

Exercise regularly

Regular exercise is essential if you want to reduce or prevent inflammation. For the best results, try to exercise every single day. Vary your workout routines and try to have fun with it! If you don't feel motivated to exercise on your own, you can try joining a class whether online or in a gym where you can work out with other people. If exercise isn't part of your current lifestyle, you can start gradually by adding more physical activities to your day such as walking to work, taking the stairs instead of the elevator, or even walking around the office every 30 minutes of sitting at your desk.

Learn how to manage your stress

I have already mentioned how stress can either cause or contribute to chronic inflammation. You want to avoid high levels of stress, and you can do this by learning how to manage your stress more effectively. There are many ways to do this such as learning time management, meditation, biofeedback, or yoga. Try out different methods to see which one works best for you.

Achieve a healthy weight

People who are either obese or overweight are more prone to inflammation. If you know that you fall into these categories, I have great news for you! By following the recommendations specified in this book and sticking with this diet, you may start shedding those stubborn excess pounds. Since this diet is healthy and balanced, your body will happily get rid of unnecessary stores that typically come in the form of excess fat and water. When you start losing weight, you can also decrease the inflammation in your body—and the risks associated with it.

Consider fasting

Have you ever considered following the intermittent fasting (IF) eating pattern? Fasting can be very beneficial in terms of reducing inflammation. And the great thing about IF is that there are several ways to do it. Pairing intermittent fasting with the anti-inflammatory diet can bring about wonderful results. Give this a try by starting with spontaneous meal skipping and work your way toward longer fasting windows. Your body will thank you for it.

Don't allow yourself to get 'hangry'

When it comes to fasting, you should do it gradually. Otherwise, you might end up feeling 'hangry'. This is when you feel so hungry that you end up getting angry at every little thing. Although 'hangry' isn't a technical term, it perfectly describes the situation. When you're hangry, you'll tend to overeat. What's worse, you'll end up craving unhealthy foods that are typically inflammatory in nature, too.

Take an alcohol break

Since excessive consumption of alcohol can cause inflammation, you may want to take a (temporary) alcohol break. If you're the kind of person who likes having a glass of wine, a bottle of beer, or a cocktail every night, consider curbing the impulse for a couple of days. Doing this helps your body calm down while reducing any inflammation that is occurring inside your body. Then, you can go back to your routine—but this time, opt for healthier alcoholic beverages that don't contain added sugar.

Of course, if you want to reduce inflammation and improve your health in the long run, you may want to give up alcohol consumption altogether. I understand that this is one of the more difficult things to do, especially since enjoying a glass of red wine after a long, tiring day seems very relaxing, but your body will surely thank you for it! If you're still unsure, why don't you conduct an experiment? Try to take a "10 Day Challenge" where you give up alcohol and replace it with a healthier habit—like going to bed early. Do this for ten days and see how it improves your health. Then, try to keep this habit up for a longer period...

Get enough sleep each night

These days, we feel like we don't have enough time throughout the day to do everything we want or need to do. Because of this, we tend to stay up late in an attempt to finish all of our tasks on time. In some cases, people stay up because it is their only time to unwind and relax. But isn't it much more relaxing to fall asleep early? It's healthier, too. Getting enough sleep each night (between seven to eight hours) helps your body rest and repair itself. But if you routinely get fewer than the recommended hours of sleep, this can exacerbate the inflammation in your body—and it might even lead to chronic inflammation.

Be a picky eater

While being a picky eater isn't a good thing for children, as an adult, this is something you need to start practicing. Whether you are choosing ingredients for cooking or you are looking for ready-to-eat foods, it's important to check labels to make sure that you are only getting healthy items.

Choose anti-inflammatory foods

Finally, you should start following the anti-inflammatory diet. This is a very easy diet as it isn't too strict or restrictive. You simply have to learn how to make healthier choices in terms of food and follow a couple of simple guidelines to make you healthier. For instance, you'll have to load up on fruits and veggies, flavor your meals with herbs and spices, introduce probiotics into your diet, minimize your consumption of dairy, and make a few more adjustments to "clean up" your existing diet.

With all of these tips in mind, you are now ready to learn more about the anti-inflammatory diet. Among all of the lifestyle changes you need to make, this is probably the most significant one—so keep reading!

The Principles of the Anti-Inflammatory Diet

The anti-inflammatory diet doesn't just reduce or prevent inflammation; the very nature of this diet promotes long-term health. By lowering inflammation in your body, you can also lower your risk of developing other diseases. This even helps slow down the aging process while increasing your metabolism, too. Although this diet doesn't come with strict rules, it does have a couple of principles to guide you as you follow the anti-inflammatory eating style. Here are the basic principles of this diet:

- Consume a lot of foods that are rich in omega-3 fatty acids, such as oily fish. Eat oily fish at least three times each week.
- Eat a lot of fruits, veggies, and whole grains. These contain fiber, vitamins, minerals, and antioxidants that calm your body and help prevent inflammation.
- Opt for oils that contain healthy fats for cooking or adding flavor to your dishes.
- When cooking, flavor your dishes using natural ingredients like herbs, spices, and natural sweeteners.
- Snacking is okay, as long as you snack on anti-inflammatory options.
- Reduce your consumption of dairy products except for kefir, yogurt, or anything fermented.
- Minimize your intake of sugar (especially refined sugar) and refined carbs like white rice or white bread, for example.
- Eliminate trans fats from your diet. This means you should stay away from any foods that contain trans fats in their list of ingredients.
- Try to avoid processed foods as much as possible as these contain ingredients that cause inflammation. Over time, try to eliminate these from your diet altogether and replace these with whole, natural foods.

As you can see, the principles of the anti-inflammatory diet are very simple. Even if you plan to shift to a different type of diet sometime in the future, these principles will give you a great head start. And if you choose to remain on the anti-inflammatory diet long-term, you can be sure that your health will improve over time as your body repairs itself and starts learning how to use inflammation efficiently and only as needed.

Basic Diet Guidelines

Another great thing about this diet is that you can easily follow it, as long as you're familiar with its principles—the basic diet guidelines are based on these principles. To help you understand them, let's discuss each of these guidelines briefly.

Eat more plants

Plants such as fruits, vegetables, herbs, and spices should be your main focus on this diet. These contain vitamins, minerals, essential nutrients, and a ton of antioxidants and phytonutrients—and all of these offer anti-inflammatory benefits. Going on this diet doesn't mean that you should give up meat, but it would be better for you in the long run to learn how to eat more plants, preferably at every meal.

For centuries, plants have been used to treat various diseases, many of which are associated with inflammation. These plant-based remedies and medications have been so effective that they are still being used until today. With this in mind, imagine how healthy you will be if you make these plants part of your regular diet. You can eat them raw, add them to your dishes, or even have them for your snacks. No matter how you add plants to your diet, these nutritious foods will help reduce or prevent inflammation in your body.

Eat ancient and whole grains

Ancient grains are a type of grain that have only undergone minimal changes over time through selective breeding, compared to other grains like rice, corn, and some wheat varieties that have changed significantly. Because of this, ancient grains are believed to be healthier than modern varieties. Some examples of ancient grains are farro, spelt, sorghum, oats, barley, chia, amaranth, and buckwheat.

Whole grains are a type of grain that contain bran, germ, and endosperm, unlike refined grains that only contain endosperm. These grains are also considered healthier as they also contain more fiber. Some examples of whole grains are brown rice, barley, and rye (although these last two should be avoided if you suffer from celiac disease or gluten intolerance). Adding these grains to your diet is essential as they are rich in nutrients, antioxidants, and other substances that have anti-inflammatory properties.

Eat healthy fats

Healthy fat sources like walnuts, olive oil, avocados, salmon, and other fatty fish contain omega-3s and omega-6s—components that are known to be anti-inflammatory. Since the body cannot produce these essential fatty acids on its own, you should get them from your diet. Fortunately, there are many delicious ways you can add healthy fats to your diet to reduce inflammation in your body.

Eat nuts and seeds

Aside from chia seeds and walnuts, which contain healthy fats, other types of nuts and seeds belong in your diet, too. These contain monounsaturated and polyunsaturated fats, which can help lower your cholesterol levels. They also contain omega-3s—which, as you know, offer anti-inflammatory benefits. Some types of nuts contain vitamin E and l-arginine, as well, which can help keep inflammation at bay. Just try to avoid overindulging, especially when you eat these as a snack.

For instance, since the daily recommended value of nuts is between 30 and 60 grams, you should only eat around 5 to 10 walnuts. It's a good idea to measure an appropriate serving of nuts into a small bowl or plate instead of snacking directly from a bag or bottle of nuts. Also, remember that some types of nuts may cause inflammation due to an allergic reaction. Varieties of tree nuts like almonds, pecans, cashews, and hazelnuts, for example, can cause allergic reactions in some people—so you should first do a bit of trial-and-error to determine how different varieties affect you.

Add flavor with herbs and spices

Rather than adding too much sugar or salt to your dishes, opt for herbs and spices to make your food more flavorful. These plants typically contain a wide range of beneficial nutrients, many of which are anti-inflammatory. Some of the best herbs and spices to use are ginger, turmeric, and garlic. These are considered anti-inflammatory powerhouses, and adding them to your meals will make your culinary masterpieces more flavorful.

Support your microbiome

To do this, you need to eat foods that contain probiotics. These are considered "good bacteria" and they help lower the inflammation levels in your body. Supporting your microbiome is even more important when you suffer from inflammatory diseases, as probiotics can help improve the effects of your treatment.

Eat fewer processed foods

Processed foods are commonly associated with obesity and many chronic diseases. These are considered high GI foods that tend to stimulate inflammation in the body. To follow the anti-inflammatory diet, you need to gradually wean yourself off these types of food. Remember that this diet is clean and natural. By eliminating processed foods, you can help reduce inflammation in your body, along with the amount of damage caused by the free radicals that these foods also contain.

Consume less meat

Although lean meat is okay in moderation, you should try to limit your consumption of red meat and processed meat products. These contain saturated fats, which are known to cause inflammation, too. If you're a meat lover, try to learn how to whip up dishes that will help you overcome your meat cravings without completely restricting yourself. Once in a while, you may consume red meat, especially while you are transitioning to the anti-inflammatory diet.

Relax!

High levels of stress or prolonged stress can result in an overproduction of cortisol. When this happens, your body's ability to regulate its immune and inflammatory responses loses its effectiveness. Aside from your diet, you may want to learn how to manage your stress more effectively. Pair this with a healthier, cleaner diet, and you will surely start feeling better.

Being Smart With Your Dietary Choices

Inflammation is one of the most common factors that causes or contributes to the development of chronic diseases. Fortunately, you can reduce your risk of inflammation by making smarter and healthier diet choices. When it comes to inflammation, the foods that you eat can make a significant difference. By choosing your food wisely—which means choosing anti-inflammatory foods and avoiding foods that promote inflammation—you can avoid inflammation and all of the dangers that come with it. Nourishing your body with anti-inflammatory foods gives your immune system all of the resources it needs so that it can function well and keep chronic illnesses at bay.

By learning which foods prevent inflammation, you can be more focused on consuming nutrients that will support your health and healing. These foods won't cause inflammation in your body, which means that your body won't have to spend so much energy repairing itself. Following an anti-inflammatory diet can be simple as long as you ease into it. If you discover that you have been eating inflammatory foods, don't worry about it. After learning which foods promote inflammation and which ones help you prevent it, you can start making gradual changes to your diet. Keep adding anti-inflammatory foods and eliminating inflammatory foods until you have fully transitioned to the anti-inflammatory diet.

Foods That Fight Inflammation

Foods that fight inflammation are also called anti-inflammatory foods. Naturally, these are the ones that reduce inflammation in your body. Generally, these foods contain important nutrients like polyphenols, antioxidants, and other anti-inflammatory compounds that help make you healthier while providing protective effects, too. The anti-inflammatory foods to focus on are:

Eggs *

Eggs are considered a "functional food," as these contain essential components and nutrients that affect the body's inflammation responses. In particular, the vitamin D content of eggs makes it an amazing anti-inflammatory option.

Fish and shellfish

Fish and shellfish are wonderful sources of protein. They also contain essential nutrients like omega-3 fatty acids that help reduce inflammation. When choosing fish, it's best to opt for wild-caught instead of farm-raised. Of course, the latter is still a better option than foods that promote inflammation. You should aim to eat fish and shellfish at least three times each week. Here are some of the options you can choose from:

- Anchovies
- Herring
- Mackerel
- Oysters
- Salmon
- Sardines
- Trout
- Tuna

Fruits

Fruits are essential to your health. Considered as "nature's candy," fruits are delicious, refreshing, and they contain so many nutrients that can help prevent inflammation. For instance, avocados are rich in vitamin E and monounsaturated fats, both of which have anti-inflammatory benefits. Berries are chock-full of vitamins, minerals, fiber, and anthocyanins, a type of antioxidant that offers anti-inflammatory effects. The best types of berries to munch on are blackberries, blueberries, and raspberries.

Then, there are cherries—a delicious fruit that contains catechins and anthocyanins, antioxidants that combat inflammation. Tart cherries are best, if you're looking to reduce inflammation. Grapes are highly anti-inflammatory, too, because they also contain anthocyanins. They also contain resveratrol, a compound that offers several health benefits. Aside from these, here are more examples of fruits to include in your diet:

- Apples
- Apricots

- Bananas
- Oranges
- Pineapple
- Strawberries

Healthy fats

Using healthy fats in your cooking is a great way to include anti-inflammatory foods in your diet. Healthy fats contain omega-9 fatty acids that help reduce inflammation. Using these oils for salad dressings, cooking, and even baking can help you improve your health. Include these healthy fats in your diet:

- Avocado oil
- Coconut oil
- Grapeseed oil
- Olive oil

Herbs and spices

Herbs and spices are important additions to your diet, as they add nutrients and flavor to your dishes. When cooking various recipes, you can add these herbs and spices for a boost of anti-inflammatory goodness. For instance, garlic is very frequently used in dishes because of the flavor and aroma it brings. But aside from this, it also offers anti-inflammatory and other benefits to your health. Onions are very common, too, as they reduce inflammation, cholesterol levels, and your risk of developing heart disease.

Turmeric is one of the more exotic spices out there and it has a very strong and earthy flavor. It is typically used in Indian dishes like curries. This spice contains a potent compound known as curcumin, which helps reduce inflammation in a big way. Various herbs also reduce inflammation while adding wonderful new flavors to your dishes. As you become a great cook, experiment with the use of herbs and spices to enhance your dishes. Here are examples of herbs and spices to include in your diet:

- Cinnamon
- Cloves

- Ginger
- Rosemary
- Sage
- Thyme

Lean meat (or white meat)

If you are a fan of meat, you don't have to eliminate this completely from your diet. However, you should opt for lean, high-quality meats whenever possible. Also, choose pasture-raised, wild, grass-fed meats to avoid the compounds in meat that tend to cause inflammation in the body.

Legumes, nuts, and seeds *

Nuts and seeds contain omega-3 fatty acids, which offer anti-inflammatory benefits. Certain legumes, like beans, also offer these benefits, along with being a good source of protein. Include these legumes, nuts, and seeds in your diet:

- Almonds
- Flax
- Hazelnuts
- Kidney beans
- Navy beans
- Pistachios
- Soybeans
- Sunflower seeds
- Walnuts

Organ meats

Although red meat isn't recommended on the anti-inflammatory diet (more on this in the next section), organ meats and offal are more accepted. In fact, the more you can eat, the better! You should also try foods that are rich in glycine such as skin, joints, connective tissues, and bone broth, as these contain nutrients that may help reduce inflammation.

Probiotics

Usually, foods that are rich in probiotics come in fermented form. While some people may not appreciate the taste of these types of foods, you should include them in your diet if you want to prevent inflammation. Here are examples of probiotic-rich foods to include in your diet:

- Coconut milk kefir
- Coconut milk yogurt
- Fermented fruit
- Fermented vegetables
- Kombucha
- Water kefir

Vegetables

Just like fruits, vegetables are an essential part of any diet, even the anti-inflammatory diet. Veggies can be eaten raw or cooked, and they come in a wide range of options. Each type of vegetable has its own nutrients that help fight inflammation while providing other benefits to your health, too. For instance, broccoli is a type of cruciferous vegetable that is extremely nutrient-dense and contains antioxidants to reduce inflammation.

Mushrooms are also an amazing addition to your dishes and they come in different varieties, like portobello, shiitake, and truffles, for example. They contain antioxidants and phenols that protect your body from inflammation. Peppers, like chili and capsicum, are great, too—full of antioxidants like vitamin C that offer powerful anti-inflammatory benefits. If you want to start making healthier diet choices, include plenty of vegetables in your meals. Aim for up to eight servings of veggies like these each week:

- Acorn squash
- Arugula
- Beets
- Brussels sprouts

- Cabbage
- Carrots
- Cassava
- Cauliflower
- Celery leaves
- Collards
- Fennel
- Kale
- Leeks
- Lettuce
- Mustard greens
- Okra
- Parsnip
- Rutabaga
- Scallions
- Sea vegetables
- Spaghetti squash
- Spinach
- Sweet potato
- Turnips
- Watercress
- Winter squash

Whole grains *

Whole grains provide you with nutritious fiber. Since fiber may help reduce inflammation, you can include whole grains in your diet, too.

- Barley

- Brown rice
- Bulgur
- Oatmeal
- Quinoa
- Whole-wheat flour

However, it's important to note that some grains such as wheat, barley, and rye aren't suitable for those who suffer from gluten-intolerance or celiac disease (more on this in the next section).

Other foods and beverages

There are other types of food that don't fall into the categories above but can still fit into your diet. These include:

- Cocoa and dark chocolate contain flavanols, compounds with anti-inflammatory properties. You can use these in various recipes to make them more decadent and beneficial.
- Coffee is a beverage that contains anti-inflammatory compounds like polyphenols. If you plan to change your diet, you won't have to say goodbye to your morning cup of joe.
- Tea, especially green tea, also contains antioxidants and other healthy compounds that combat inflammation. Add lemon or honey to your tea to make it more flavorful.

When it comes to choosing anti-inflammatory foods, try to find high-quality ingredients as these won't contain any unnecessary additives that might give you the opposite effects. To keep yourself interested in anti-inflammatory foods, vary your diet as much as possible. Learning how to cook and trying various recipes will help you succeed in your anti-inflammatory diet journey.

Foods That Make Inflammation Worse

Naturally, if there are foods that help you prevent inflammation, there are also foods on the opposite side of the spectrum—the ones that make inflammation worse. Most of these foods are generally unhealthy, anyway, so it's best to eliminate them from your diet. However, you might be surprised to find some common types of food, which may offer some health benefits, also promote inflammation. To make things clearer for you, inflammatory foods to avoid are:

Alcoholic beverages (in excess)

Moderate consumption of alcohol isn't harmful—in fact, it can even be beneficial. But drinking in excess can cause a lot of problems, one of which is inflammation. The main issue with this is that excessive alcohol may cause issues with bacterial toxins that move out of your colon and into your body. This condition, known as "leaky gut," causes inflammation throughout the body. If you want to avoid this, make sure to limit your alcohol consumption to healthy levels.

Artificial trans fats

This type of fat is probably the unhealthiest one out there. If you read ingredient lists of food products, you may see this ingredient included as "partially hydrogenated oils." Artificial trans fats are typically added to processed foods for the purpose of extending their shelf life. Unfortunately, consuming this ingredient increases your risk of inflammation. Some examples of foods that may contain artificial trans fats are:

- Any processed food product that contains partially hydrogenated oil
- French fries
- Fried fast food
- Margarine (some varieties)
- Microwave popcorn (some varieties)
- Packaged cakes
- Packaged cookies
- Packaged pastries
- Vegetable shortenings

Dairy products

Generally, dairy products like milk and cheese contain high amounts of saturated fats, which can increase your risk of inflammation. This is especially true for full-fat dairy products. In some cases, severe or chronic inflammation might even cause lactose intolerance.

Nightshades *

Although nightshades are very nutritious, they can potentially cause inflammation, too. The main reason for this is the solanine content. This is a type of chemical that may aggravate inflammation in the body. Some examples of nightshades are:

- Cayenne
- Eggplants
- Goji berries
- Paprika
- Potatoes (except sweet potatoes)
- Tomatillos

Refined carbohydrates

When refined carbohydrates are processed, most of the fiber they contain is removed. This type of carbohydrate tends to increase inflammation in the body along with blood sugar levels. Some examples of foods that contain refined carbs are:

- All types of processed foods that contain added flour or sugar
- Bread
- Cakes
- Candy
- Cookies
- Cereals (some varieties)
- Pasta
- Pastries
- Soft drinks

Some types of grains

Generally, grains don't cause inflammation. But wheat, barley, and rye are grains that contain gluten, which can lead to inflammation in people with celiac disease, a wheat allergy, or non-celiac gluten sensitivity. If you suffer from any of these conditions, you should avoid these grains. Otherwise, you don't have to eliminate these from your diet.

Sugar

High-fructose corn syrup and table sugar don't belong in your diet, as they increase inflammation, too. Unfortunately, so many food products contain these ingredients, so you have to be very careful when buying sweet treats. Some examples of foods that contain added sugar are:

- Candy
- Cakes
- Cereals (some varieties)
- Chocolate

- Cookies
- Doughnuts
- Soft drinks
- Sweet pastries

Processed and red meat

Although lean meat is okay in moderation, red meat and processed meat products are huge no-nos. These foods increase your risk of inflammation along with a number of chronic diseases, too. Processed meats also contain high amounts of advanced glycation end-products, which are known to drive inflammation. Some examples of processed and red meats are:

- Bacon
- Beef jerky
- Burgers
- Canned meat
- Hot dogs
- Sausages
- Salami
- Smoked meat
- Steaks
- Ham

Vegetable oils

Vegetables belong in your diet, but oils derived from vegetables are another story. Since most vegetable oils are highly processed, they usually contain excessive omega-6 amounts. Unhealthy amounts of this fatty acid can cause inflammation, especially if you suffer from inflammatory conditions like irritable bowel syndrome or arthritis.

Other inflammatory foods

There are other types of food that don't fall into the categories above but can still cause inflammation. These include:

- Artificial sweeteners
- Convenience meals
- Egg rolls
- Energy drinks
- Foods that are high in sodium, like potato chips and other junk foods
- Fried chicken
- Mozzarella sticks
- Pretzels
- Sports drinks
- Sweet tea

As you may have noticed, several of these foods appear in more than one category. This indicates that such foods truly are inflammatory and you should stay away from them as much as possible.

Foods That are Both Inflammatory and Anti-Inflammatory

As you familiarize yourself with these food lists and start planning your meals, you should know there are certain foods that may have both inflammatory and anti-inflammatory effects. You may have noticed some foods in the anti-inflammatory list that have asterisks—these are the foods to look out for.

Eggs

Eggs are extremely healthy, but they do affect people in various ways. Factors like existing diseases and a person's weight can have an impact on whether or not eggs will cause inflammation in the body. This is especially true for egg whites. Because of this, you have to observe your body right after eating eggs to check if you experience any negative effects, which may indicate inflammation.

If you discover that eggs don't agree with you, you can use egg replacements in recipes that call for this ingredient. There are commercial egg replacers you can use, like vegan liquid egg yolks, and you can also make your own egg replacers in your own kitchen. If you prefer homemade options, you can use tofu, aquafaba (plain cooking brine from chickpeas), or even fruits like bananas, or squash. Check your local health food stores for these healthy substitutes so you can continue creating delicious recipes even if they contain eggs.

Legumes, nuts, and seeds

Probably the riskiest legume you can eat in terms of inflammation is peanuts. Although peanuts are very common, they contain a family of toxins known as aflatoxins, which can potentially stimulate an inflammatory response in your body. For other legumes, the inflammatory effect may come from their lectin content. Since lectins are hard for the body to break down, this may cause inflammation. Aside from legumes, other examples of nuts and seeds that may cause inflammation are:

- Nut butters
- Nut flours
- Nut oils
- Seed-based spices
- Seed oil

Nightshades

When it comes to inflammation, one of the most commonly avoided types of veggies are nightshades. In the last section, we discussed the reason for this. But it's also important to note that the most commonly consumed nightshades contain minimal amounts of solanine, the compound that triggers inflammation. However, newer research shows that these vegetables are, in fact, okay to consume—and some even contain powerful nutrients that offer anti-inflammatory benefits.

For instance, one study published in a medical journal showed that potatoes, peppers, tomatoes, and eggplants contain an alkaloid compound that has very potent anti-inflammatory effects (Lanier, R., et. al., 2013). This means that these nightshades can be beneficial and even ideal for the anti-inflammatory diet. Some people might have a sensitivity to these nightshades, but not all of them are inherently inflammatory.

Consider tomatoes, which are part of the nightshade family. Most people believe that they are inflammatory because tomatoes, like other nightshades, contain solanine. But aside from the fact that tomatoes don't contain high levels of the chemical, it also doesn't affect all people the same way. While some people might experience inflammatory effects, this may not apply to you. By eliminating tomatoes from your diet, you will be missing out on their wonderful lycopene and vitamin C contents, both of which provide powerful antioxidant and anti-inflammatory properties.

For tomatoes and other nightshade veggies, you will have to observe yourself after consuming them. If they trigger symptoms of inflammation, then nightshades might not be right for you. If not, you can continue eating them and adding them to your dishes. As you will see in the upcoming recipes, some of them do contain nightshades. If these veggies trigger inflammation in your body, you can either skip the ingredients or replace them. For instance, potatoes can be replaced with sweet potatoes, tomatoes with olives (or simply removed from the recipe), or peppers with carrots (you can remove these, too). Remember, it's all about finding what works best for you as you improve your health through the anti-inflammatory diet.

The key to determining whether to eat or avoid any of these foods is observation. As you eliminate inflammatory foods from your diet, you will start seeing positive changes in your health. When you consume these foods, pay attention to your body to see how you react to them. Aside from these "special foods", there are also certain foods that you should only eat in moderation so that they won't increase your risk of inflammation. These are:

Black tea

Blackstrap molasses

Coconut

Dried fruits

Fructose

Honey

Plantains

Poultry

Salt (when using salt, opt for unrefined varieties)

Saturated fat

Going on an anti-inflammatory diet doesn't have to feel difficult or restricting. You shouldn't deprive yourself of the foods you love, especially in the beginning. Remember, it's always best to ease into the diet to give your body the chance to adjust to the new foods you are introducing and the foods you are gradually weaning yourself from. This is the best way to learn how to make smarter and healthier food choices for the rest of your life!

CHAPTER 2: A 10-DAY MEAL PLAN FOR YOU + YOUR SHOPPING LIST GUIDE

Now that you know more about inflammation and which foods can help you become healthier, it's time to create a meal plan for yourself. In this chapter, you will learn how to make an awesome meal plan for ten days to help your body heal and become healthier. This serves as a sample to give you an idea of how to approach the whole meal-planning process. After practicing with these meals (both planning and cooking them), you can start creating your own meal plan to continue with the anti-inflammatory diet. But before we go through the 10-day meal plan, let's first discuss the common ingredients you'll want to stock up on. That way, you'll always have the right ingredients ready for when you want to start cooking your meals.

Shopping on the Anti-Inflammatory Diet

As you transition to an anti-inflammatory diet, you will have to be more conscious when choosing food items and ingredients for your meals. As much as possible, try to stick with fresh, whole ingredients instead of packaged and processed products. Of course, as you learned, there are certain whole foods that might promote inflammation in your body, too. Fortunately, we covered these in the previous chapter, so you know what to avoid or eat in moderation.

When stocking up your pantry, you don't have to buy all of these things at the same time. Start by making a list of what you need for specific recipes, and if you see common ingredients, you can buy more of these. But if you notice certain ingredients that are used sparingly and in only a few recipes, you can buy minimal quantities. This is especially true for ingredients that have a long shelf life. As you learn more recipes and get used to meal planning and cooking your own meals, your pantry will grow eventually. And when you have a pantry stocked with staples that you always use, cooking healthy anti-inflammatory meals becomes much easier. Here are some of the most common ingredients you may encounter in anti-inflammatory recipes:

Healthy oils

Opt for "expeller-pressed" or "cold-pressed" oils, as these haven't undergone heat processing that tends to compromise the quality of the oils. The best options are olive oil, extra virgin olive oil, almond oil, and coconut oil (especially for baking).

Fermented foods

Whether store-bought or homemade, fermented foods are great because they support the health of your gut. Some options to try are kombucha, yogurt, kimchi, and sauerkraut.

Flour

Opt for gluten-free flour like buckwheat, almond, coconut, or brown rice flour.

Fresh fruits and veggies

For these ingredients, choose all the colors. Whether fresh or frozen, fruits and veggies are essential for your diet. But remember that fresh fruits and veggies may spoil easily, so it's recommended to buy these right before you plan to eat them or use them in recipes.

Garlic and onion

These add nutrition and flavor to your dishes.

Ginger and turmeric

These are some of the healthiest spices you can include in your dishes to add a valuable anti-inflammatory benefit. You can put these into soups, smoothies, dressings, curries, and other amazing dishes.

Grains

Choose gluten-free varieties like quinoa, amaranth, or brown rice. Gluten-free oats are a good choice, too.

Herbs and spices

Whether fresh or dried, herbs and spices give your dishes more flavor and a boost of nutrition. Apart from offering an anti-inflammatory effect, these ingredients come with their own unique health benefits.

Legumes

Be careful when choosing nuts and seeds, as some may promote inflammation. Opt for legumes that have anti-inflammatory benefits like lentils, kidney beans, garbanzo beans, or black beans.

Limes and lemons

You can use these for cooking, or try slicing them and adding the slices to water to make it healthier and more flavorful.

Natural sweeteners

To avoid inflammation, you should only use these in moderation. Some of the best types of natural sweeteners are pure maple syrup, brown rice syrup, dates, or agave syrup.

Nuts and seeds

Be careful when choosing nuts and seeds as some may promote inflammation. Try to see how your body reacts whenever you eat them, before you use them in your dishes or eat them as a snack. Generally, though, some of the healthiest nuts are almonds, pecans, cashews, and walnuts. For seeds, the best options are pumpkin, hemp, flax, and chia seeds.

Sea salt

Opt for unrefined, as the refined variety doesn't contain minerals. Pink or gray sea salt are amazing options.

Tea and coffee

If possible, take your tea and coffee plain. This allows you to get all of their health benefits without adding sugar or dairy to the mix. For tea, some great options are rooibos, white, holy basil, and green tea.

Vinegar

Vinegar can be used for cooking and it's an excellent option for salad dressings. Some of the best types are apple cider, white wine, or balsamic vinegar.

If you have all of these basics in your kitchen, cooking becomes much easier and more convenient for you. For instance, even if you miss out buying a specific ingredient from your weekly grocery list, you likely already have it in your pantry—or at least a good alternative for it. Just make sure to check your refrigerator and pantry before meal planning or creating a shopping list. That way, you won't have to buy ingredients that you already have and you can include your leftovers in your plan. Part of becoming an efficient meal planner is learning how to reduce food waste while following a clean, healthy, anti-inflammatory diet.

With all of these basics in mind, let's create a meal plan for your first ten days as you transition into a new diet that focuses on anti-inflammatory foods. This is a sample meal plan that comes with a daily shopping list. When you reach the end of this chapter, try to come up with an organized list of all the needed ingredients that you can bring to the supermarket. Then, you can start cooking by following the simple recipes in the next three chapters.

Day 1

For Day 1, here are some sample meals you can whip up for yourself, followed by a sample list of ingredients for you to make those meals. You can add the quantities after checking the recipes (in the next three chapters) and doing an inventory of your pantry and kitchen.

Meal Plan

- **Breakfast**: Wake-Me-Up Salad
- **Lunch**: Orange Chicken and Vegetables
- **Dinner**: Low-Carb Rice Bowl

Shopping List

For the recipes above, you will need the following ingredients:

apples

arugula

avocado oil

baby spinach

beets

black pepper

blueberries

chicken broth

chicken thighs

dried oregano

extra virgin olive oil

garlic

green cabbage

ground ginger

ground turkey

kale

orange

persimmon

red radish

mushrooms

sea salt

sweet potatoes

tarragon

walnuts

yellow onion

zucchini squash

Day 2

These meals are tasty, easy, and varied. Here you'll find the list of ingredients needed to make these meals, and in the next three chapters, you can check the quantities each recipe calls for.

Meal Plan

- **Breakfast**: Blueberry Smoothie with Hemp Seeds
- **Lunch**: Oven-Baked Tilapia
- **Dinner**: Chicken and Veggie Stir-Fry

Shopping List

For the recipes above, you will need the following ingredients:

black pepper

chicken breasts

chlorella powder

cilantro

coconut palm sugar

cooking spray

egg (or store-bought egg replacers)

frozen blueberries

garlic

hemp seeds

olive oil

plant-based milk (unsweetened)

plant-based protein powder (vanilla flavor)

raw pecans

red bell pepper

rice vinegar

rosemary

salt

scallions

sesame seeds

snap peas

soy sauce

spinach

tilapia fillets

whole-wheat breadcrumbs

Day 3

For Day 3, you have a blend of hearty, healthy, sweet, and savory dishes to enjoy from morning until night. Don't forget to check the quantities of the ingredients to buy, as well as your own stocks before you head to the supermarket.

Meal Plan

- **Breakfast**: Sweet and Savory Breakfast Hash
- **Lunch**: Beef and Veggie Skillet
- **Dinner**: Hearty Detox Salad

Shopping List

For the recipes above, you will need the following ingredients:

apple

avocado

avocado oil

baby kale

broccoli

butternut squash

carrots

cinnamon

coconut oil

dried thyme

garlic powder

ginger

green onion

ground beef

ground turkey

lemon

maple syrup

onion

parsley

powdered ginger

radishes

raw almonds

red bell pepper

red cabbage

sea salt

spinach

stone-ground mustard

turmeric

yellow squash

zucchini

zucchini squash

Day 4

These meals are quick, interesting, and quite unique. The lunch and dinner recipes here also happen to be highly customizable, which means that you can mix and match the ingredients according to your preferences. Just make sure to update your shopping list when you make changes to the recipes.

Meal Plan

- **Breakfast**: 5-Minute Avocado Toast
- **Lunch**: Charred Shrimp Buddha Bowl
- **Dinner**: Pineapple Sweetened Fried Rice

Shopping List

For the recipes above, you will need the following ingredients:

arugula

avocado

balsamic vinegar

black pepper

brown rice

carrots

celery

cherry tomatoes

eggs (or store-bought egg replacers)

extra virgin olive oil

frozen corn

frozen peas

garlic

green onion

ham

lemons

olive oil

onion

pesto

pineapple (canned or fresh)

powdered ginger

quinoa

salt

sesame oil

shrimps

soy sauce

white pepper

whole-wheat toast

Day 5

For Day 5, you will enjoy savory dishes that are all healthy and filling. By this time, you will already be getting used to the diet, which is good news for you! Just keep going… you're halfway through your anti-inflammatory meal plan!

Meal Plan

- **Breakfast**: Creamy Whole-Grain Breakfast Porridge
- **Lunch**: Silky Avocado Pesto
- **Dinner**: Mediterranean-Style Cod

Shopping List

For the recipes above, you will need the following ingredients:

almond milk

apple

avocados

basil

black pepper

capers

cherry tomatoes

chia seeds

cinnamon

cod fillets

cooking spray

dates

extra virgin olive oil

garlic

garlic powder

lemons

nutmeg

olive oil

oregano

paprika

pasta

pine nuts

quinoa

raw honey

raw walnuts

ripe olives

salt

sea salt

sunflower seeds

thyme

walnuts

Day 6

On Day 6, you will focus on different types of veggies cooked in different ways. As you can see, adding more vegetables to your diet can make your meals tastier and more varied. Most people don't see this until they start making healthy changes to the way they eat.

Meal Plan

- **Breakfast**: Veggie Omelet
- **Lunch**: Poke Salad with Seared Tuna
- **Dinner**: Roasted Sheet Pan Veggies

Shopping List

For the recipes above, you will need the following ingredients:

ahi tuna steak

arugula

asparagus

avocado

black pepper

cherry tomatoes

cilantro

cooking spray

cornstarch

eggs (store-bought egg replacers)

feta cheese

garlic

ginger

honey

jalapeño

Kalamata olives

lime

olive oil

pineapple

pineapple juice

rice vinegar

salt

sesame seeds

Sriracha

soy sauce

spring greens

tahini

toasted sesame oil

tomatoes

thyme

wonton wrappers

Day 7

For Day 7, you will notice that these recipes have different flavors and textures. These meals will tantalize your taste buds to make you feel more convinced of the long-term sustainability of this healthy diet.

Meal Plan

- **Breakfast**: Chia Pudding with Hemp
- **Lunch**: Skillet-Cooked Salmon
- **Dinner**: Refreshing Salad with Crunchy Chickpeas

Shopping List

For the recipes above, you will need the following ingredients:

avocado oil

black pepper

capers

cardamom

cherry tomatoes

chia seeds

chickpeas

coconut milk

coriander

cumin

dates

dried dill

garlic

ground cinnamon

ground ginger

hemp seeds

hummus

lemon

lettuce

olive oil

paprika

parsley

plant-based milk (unsweetened)

quinoa

raw cacao powder

red onion

salmon

sea salt

smoked paprika

turmeric

sea salt

water

Day 8

For Day 8, treat yourself to unique cuisines by whipping up new and unfamiliar dishes. Don't worry, though, these are super easy to make, too. And once you start eating, you will enjoy this diet even more!

Meal Plan

- **Breakfast**: Anti-Inflammatory Shakshuka
- **Lunch**: Greek-Style Turkey Burgers
- **Dinner**: Fresh and Healthy Shrimp Wrap

Shopping List

For the recipes above, you will need the following ingredients:

avocado

black pepper

Boston lettuce

cherry tomatoes

cilantro

cooking spray

coriander

dried cumin

dried oregano

eggs (or store-bought egg replacers)

European cucumber

extra virgin olive oil

feta cheese

garlic

garlic powder

Greek yogurt

ground turkey

harissa

jalapeño

lemon

lime

onion

parsley

red onion

red pepper flakes

salt

scallion

shrimp

spinach

sweet onion

tomato

vegetable broth

whole-wheat bread crumbs

whole-wheat hamburger buns

whole-wheat tortilla wrap

Day 9

On Day 9, you will be cooking your meals in different ways. By this time, you may already have some leftover ingredients from previous days. Don't forget to take an inventory of your kitchen or pantry before you start shopping. This ensures you won't have a lot of food waste, especially in terms of fresh produce.

Meal Plan

- **Breakfast**: Healthy Chickpea Scramble Stuffed Sweet Potatoes
- **Lunch**: Anti-Inflammatory Green Curry
- **Dinner**: Quinoa Salad with Salmon

Shopping List

For the recipes above, you will need the following ingredients:

avocado

avocado oil

broccoli

brown sugar

chickpeas

cilantro

coconut milk

extra virgin olive oil

firm tofu

fish sauce

garlic

green curry paste

golden raisins

kale

olive oil

onion

pepper

pistachios

quinoa

red bell peppers

red wine vinegar

salmon

salt

sea salt

sweet potatoes

turmeric

Day 10

Day 10 will be the last day of your anti-inflammatory meal plan. Now, you have to start thinking about making your own meal plan to continue with this diet. Since you've already had several examples of the types of meals to eat, you'll be able to come up with your own healthy options.

Meal Plan

- **Breakfast**: High-Protein Breakfast Bowl
- **Lunch**: Citrus Salad with Roasted Beets
- **Dinner**: Mediterranean Vegetable Wraps

Shopping List

For the recipes above, you need the following ingredients:

avocado

avocado oil

baby arugula

baby greens

baby spinach

balsamic vinegar

banana

beet

black pepper

blood orange

blueberries

chia seeds

chickpeas

cilantro

clementine

cucumber

dried oregano

feta cheese

garlic

hemp hearts

lemon

multi-grain wraps

olive oil

pistachios

plant-based protein powder

raspberries

red onion

salt

sea salt

sweet potato

tahini

tomato

white pepper

CHAPTER 3: BREAKFAST RECIPES FOR YOUR MEAL PLAN

Ah, breakfast... the most important meal of the day. As you create your meal plan, don't forget to include a healthy, filling, and tasty breakfast that will help you combat inflammation. Although some diets recommend that you skip breakfast, you don't have to do this if you can prepare nutrient-rich breakfast recipes for yourself that will help you feel satisfied and energized. In this chapter, you will learn such recipes. As you will see, all of these dishes fit into the meal plan from the last chapter. Of course, you can mix and match these recipes to create your own meal plan that you will be happy with.

Wake-Me-Up Salad

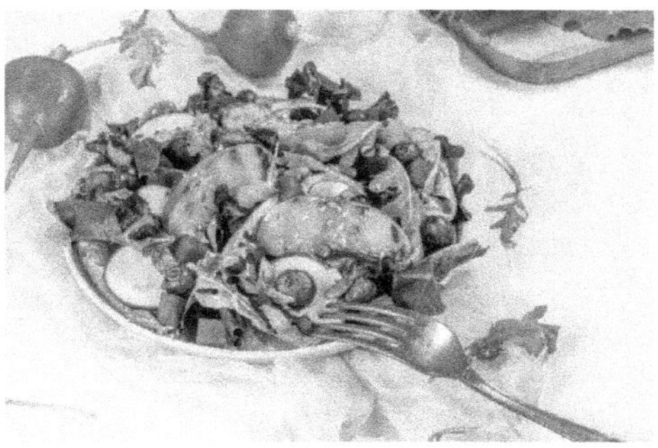

When you wake up in the morning, you need a burst of energy—and you get this from your first meal of the day. Although salads are healthy by nature, you don't have to settle for boring salads that only include a couple of tasteless ingredients. Here is one example of an amazing salad (there's more to come!) that will make you feel energized, satisfied, and happy. Aside from being anti-inflammatory, this salad is vegan and gluten-free, too!

Time: 10 minutes

Serving Size: 2 servings

Prep Time: 10 minutes

Cook Time: no cooking time

Ingredients for the salad:

- ¼ cup of walnuts (chopped, you can use other nuts)
- ¾ cup of blueberries (fresh)
- 3 red radishes (thinly sliced)
- 1 persimmon (chopped)
- 1 cup of beets (cooked, peeled, cooled, chopped)
- ½ cup of arugula
- ½ cup of spring mix lettuce (rinsed, chopped)

Ingredients for the dressing:

- ½ tsp ginger (freshly grated)
- ½ tsp turmeric
- ½ tbsp lemon juice (freshly squeezed)
- 1 tbsp apple cider vinegar
- ¼ cup of extra virgin olive oil
- ½ clove of garlic (grated)
- Black pepper
- Salt

Directions:

1. In a bowl, add all of the dressing ingredients and mix until well incorporated.
2. Divide the salad ingredients between 2 serving bowls.
3. Drizzle with dressing and toss lightly to coat.
4. Serve immediately for a refreshingly healthy breakfast.

Blueberry Smoothie with Hemp Seeds

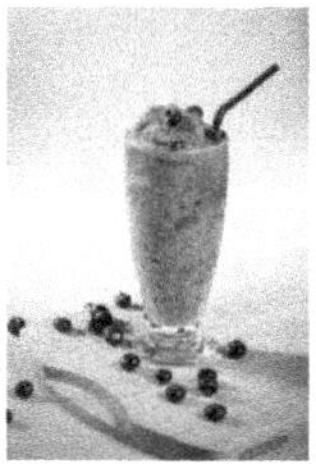

Smoothies are an excellent breakfast option if you're always dealing with busy mornings—and you can easily mix and match ingredients to suit your taste. Now that you know the best anti-inflammatory foods to choose from, you can use those as ingredients for your smoothies. This recipe includes anti-inflammatory ingredients that are nourishing and satisfying. While this smoothie will give you a boost of energy in the morning, you can also enjoy it at any time of the day.

Time: 5 minutes

Serving Size: 1 smoothie

Prep Time: 5 minutes

Cook Time: no cooking time

Ingredients:

- 1 tsp chlorella powder (you can also use spirulina)
- 2 tbsp hemp seeds
- 2 tbsp plant-based protein powder (vanilla flavor)
- ½ cup of spinach (fresh, you can also use kale)
- 1 ¼ cup of blueberries (frozen, you can also use other types of frozen berries)
- 1 ¼ cup of milk (unsweetened, plant-based)

Directions:

1. In a blender, add all of the ingredients.
2. Blend on high speed until you get a creamy and smooth texture.
3. Pour the smoothie into a glass and enjoy!

Sweet and Savory Breakfast Hash

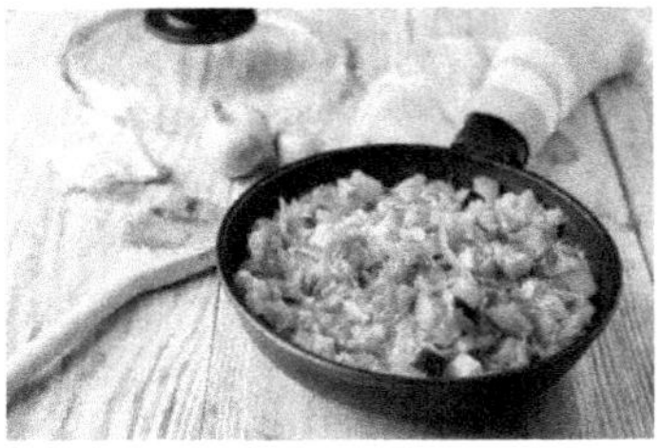

There's nothing more satisfying than a dish that has sweet and savory flavors blended together perfectly. Although some people might raise their eyebrows at this combination, trust me... it works! This is a protein-rich breakfast that's packed with turkey and anti-inflammatory veggies to keep you healthy, strong, and free of bad inflammation.

Time: 25 minutes

Serving Size: 2 servings

Prep Time: 10 minutes

Cook Time: 15 minutes

Ingredients for the turkey:

- ¼ tsp cinnamon
- ¼ tsp thyme (dried)
- ½ tbsp coconut oil
- ½ lb ground turkey
- Sea salt

Ingredients for the hash:

- ¼ tsp garlic powder
- ¼ tsp thyme (dried)
- ¼ tsp turmeric
- ⅓ tsp ginger (powdered)
- ½ tsp cinnamon

- ½ tbsp coconut oil
- ¼ cup of carrots (shredded)
- 1 cup of butternut squash (cubed, you can also use sweet potato)
- 1 cup of spinach (you can also use other types of greens)
- ½ onion (chopped)
- 1 small apple (peeled, cored, chopped)
- 1 small zucchini (chopped)
- Sea salt

Directions:

1. In a skillet, warm half of the coconut oil over medium-high heat.
2. Add the turkey and cook until it's browned.
3. While cooking, season the meat with the spices and mix well.
4. Once cooked, move the turkey onto a plate.
5. Add the remaining coconut oil into the skillet, along with the onion.
6. Sauté the onion until softened for about 2 to 3 minutes.
7. Add the apple, carrots, squash, and zucchini and cook until softened for about 4 to 5 minutes.
8. Add the spinach and continue cooking until the leaves wilt.
9. Add the cooked turkey, along with the hash seasonings, then continue mixing. Taste the hash and adjust the seasonings according to your taste.
10. Spoon the hash onto serving plates and serve immediately.

5-Minute Avocado Toast

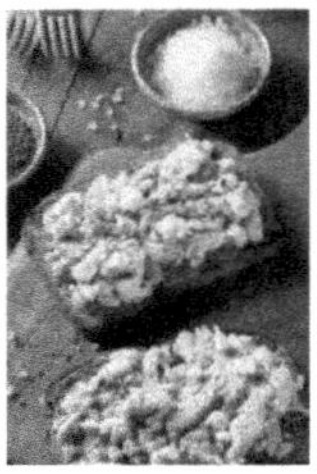

Avocado on toast is a simple, classic dish, but this recipe takes things up a notch. Basically, you will be adding egg salad to make your toast healthier and tastier. This amazing recipe only takes five minutes to make, but it will keep you full and energized all morning.

Time: 5 minutes

Serving Size: 1 serving

Prep Time: 5 minutes

Cook Time: no cooking time

Ingredients:

- ½ tsp lemon juice (freshly squeezed)
- 1 tbsp celery (chopped)
- ¼ avocado
- 1 hard-boiled egg (chopped, you can also use ⅓ cup of cubed tofu or store-bought egg replacers)
- 1 slice of toast (whole-wheat)
- Salt

Directions:

1. In a bowl, add the avocado and mash well.
2. Add the lemon juice, celery, and salt, then mix until well incorporated.
3. Fold in the egg until just combined.
4. Spread the mixture on the slice of toast. If you want it to be crunchy, toast the bread first to your desired doneness.
5. Enjoy!

Creamy Whole-Grain Breakfast Porridge

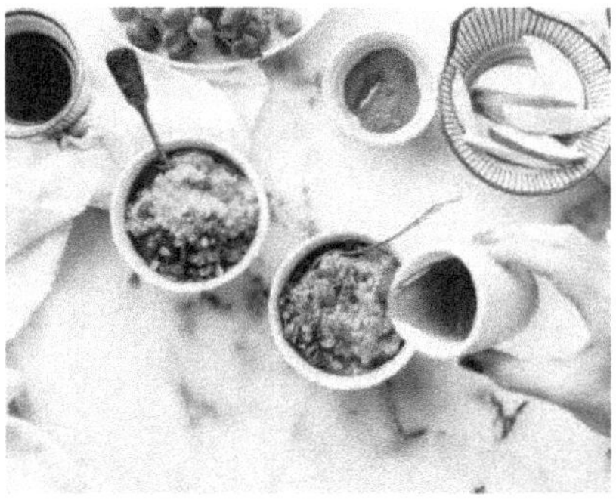

Porridge is one of the most filling dishes you can make for yourself. This quick recipe is super easy to prepare and you can customize the ingredients so you don't get bored. For instance, you can top your porridge with sweet fruits like bananas or berries, and you can add nuts or seeds for added texture. Basically, anything you want to add, you can—just make sure to stick with anti-inflammatory options.

Time: 15 minutes

Serving Size: 1 serving

Prep Time: 5 minutes

Cook Time: 10 minutes

Ingredients for the porridge:

- 1 tsp cinnamon
- 2 tbsp of dates (chopped, you can also use raisins or cranberries)
- ½ cup of quinoa (cooked, you can also use teff, brown rice, or amaranth)
- ¼ cup of raw walnuts (you can also use cashews, pecans, or almonds)
- ¼ cup of sunflower seeds (you can also use hemp seeds or pumpkin seeds)
- ¼ cup of almond milk (you can also use coconut, cashew, oat, hemp or rice milk)

Ingredients for the toppings (optional):

- 1 tbsp chia seeds (you can also use ground flax seeds)
- 1 tbsp sweetener (like raw honey, liquid stevia extract, or maple syrup)

- ½ apple (diced)
- Nutmeg (just a pinch, you can also use ginger, turmeric, cloves, or cardamom)

Directions:

1. In a saucepan, add all of the porridge ingredients over medium heat. Adjust the amount of milk until you achieve your desired consistency.
2. Continue warming the porridge until you get a creamy and soft mixture that is completely heated through.
3. Once cooked, pour the porridge into a bowl and add your desired toppings.
4. Enjoy while warm and creamy.

Veggie Omelet

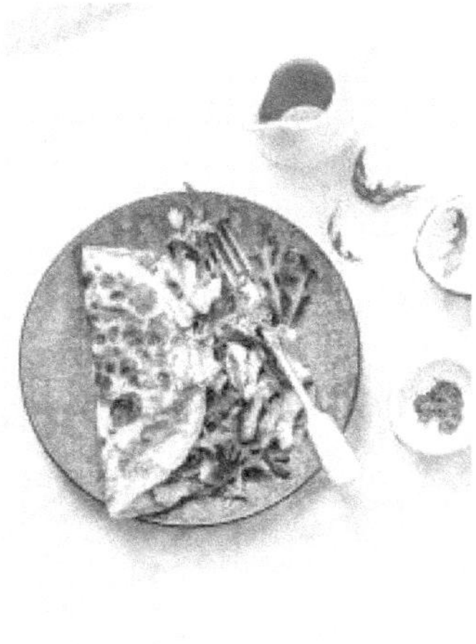

Although this recipe is simple, it comes together as an elegant breakfast dish that you will surely love to eat. It contains anti-inflammatory ingredients that are healthy, filling, and combine perfectly. This recipe takes less than half an hour to prepare, which means that you will have more time to enjoy it!

Time: 15 minutes

Serving Size: 2 servings

Prep Time: 5 minutes

Cook Time: 10 minutes

Ingredients:

- 1 avocado (sliced)
- ¼ cup of feta cheese (crumbled)
- ½ cup of arugula (fresh, you can also use spinach)
- 4 eggs (lightly beaten, you can also use silken tofu or store-bought egg replacers)
- Black pepper
- Cooking spray
- ½ cup of tomato (optional, seeded, chopped, you can also use olives instead)

Directions:

1. Grease a skillet with cooking spray and warm over medium heat.
2. In the bowl with the egg, add a pinch of pepper and mix well.
3. Pour half of the egg mixture into the skillet.
4. Using a spatula, stir the eggs continuously but gently until you get small cooked pieces of egg surrounded by uncooked liquid egg.
5. Continue cooking for another 1 minute until the egg is still shiny but has already set.
6. Add half of the veggies into the skillet on one half of the egg.
7. Use the spatula to lift the other half of the egg then fold it over to cover the veggies.
8. Gently transfer the omelet to a plate, then repeat the cooking steps to cook another omelet.
9. Serve while warm and enjoy.

Chia Pudding with Hemp

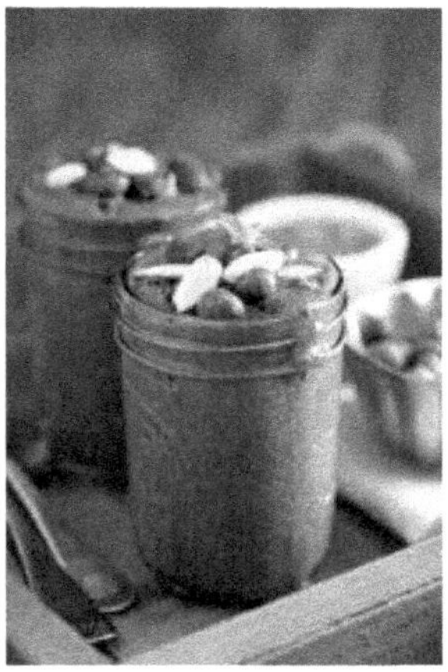

Chia pudding is quickly becoming a favorite breakfast recipe among health enthusiasts because it's tasty, easy, and super customizable. This recipe is rich in omega-3 fatty acids that fight inflammation along with fiber, antioxidants, vitamins, and minerals. This is another recipe that you can mix and match according to your tastes. You can even add more ingredients to make this pudding healthier and more filling.

Time: 5 minutes (chilling time not included)

Serving Size: 1 serving

Prep Time: 5 minutes

Cook Time: no cooking time

Ingredients:

- 1 tbsp cacao powder (raw)
- 2 tbsp chia seeds
- 2 tbsp hemp seeds
- 6 small dates (pitted)
- ½ cup of milk (unsweetened, preferably plant-based)
- ¼ tsp grey sea salt (optional)
- ½ tsp vanilla extract (optional)

- 1 tbsp protein powder (optional, chocolate flavor, preferably plant-based)

Directions:

1. In a blender, add all of the ingredients and blend until well combined.
2. Pour the mixture into a container with a lid.
3. Place the container in the refrigerator for at least 2 hours.
4. When you're ready to eat breakfast, add toppings of your choice and enjoy!

** Some suggestions for toppings are banana slices, nut butter, walnuts, berries, almonds, pumpkin seeds, or sunflower seeds.*

Anti-Inflammatory Shakshuka

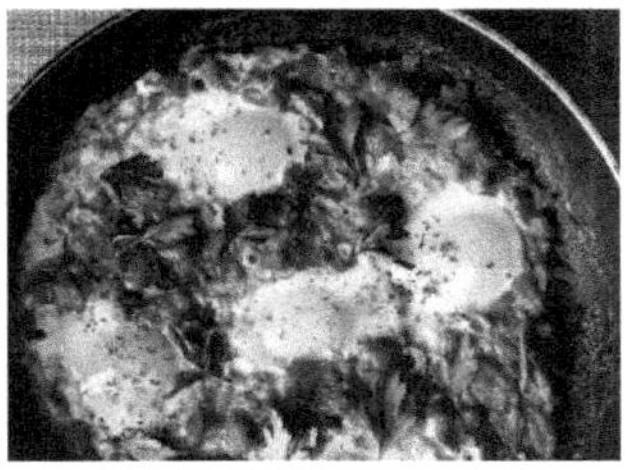

Just because you want to follow an anti-inflammatory diet, that doesn't mean you have to stick with the same old dishes every day. If you want to keep things interesting, learn how to make unique dishes that will tantalize your taste buds. This is one such dish. It looks amazingly fancy, but it's super easy to make. The best part? It tastes as good as it looks!

Time: 30 minutes

Serving Size: 2 servings

Prep Time: 5 minutes

Cook Time: 25 minutes

Ingredients:

- ¼ tsp coriander
- ½ tsp cumin (dried)
- 1 tbsp extra virgin olive oil
- 1 tbsp harissa
- ¼ cup of vegetable broth
- 2 cups of spinach
- ½ jalapeño (seeded, minced)
- ½ onion (minced)
- 1 clove of garlic (minced)
- 4 large eggs (you can also use ⅔ cup of silky tofu or store-bought egg replacers)
- Black pepper

- Cooking spray
- Salt
- Cilantro (fresh, chopped, for serving)
- Parsley (fresh, chopped, for serving)

Directions:

1. Preheat your oven to 350°F.
2. In an oven-safe skillet, add the olive oil over medium heat, along with the onions.
3. Sauté the onions for about 4 to 5 minutes until tender.
4. Add the jalapeño and garlic and continue sautéing for 1 more minute until fragrant.
5. Add the spinach and continue sautéing for about 1 to 2 minutes until wilted.
6. Season the mixture with harissa, coriander, cumin, salt, and pepper, and continue sautéing for 1 minute more to combine everything well.
7. Spoon the vegetable mixture into a blender and purée until you get a coarse texture.
8. Add the vegetable broth and continue blending until the texture becomes smooth and thick.
9. Wipe the skillet with a paper towel and use cooking spray to grease it lightly.
10. Pour the vegetable mixture into the skillet, then make 4 circle-shaped wells using a wooden spoon.
11. Carefully crack one egg into each of the wells.
12. Place the skillet in the oven and cook for about 15 to 20 minutes until the eggs are fully set.
13. Take the skillet out of the oven.
14. Sprinkle with fresh cilantro and parsley before serving.

Healthy Chickpea Scramble Stuffed Sweet Potatoes

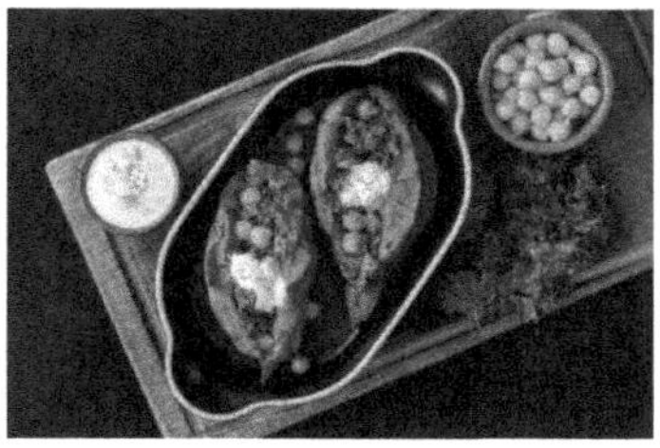

Chickpeas are healthy, nourishing, and chock-full of nutrients. This dish looks very appetizing and it tastes incredible, too. This is a plant-based recipe that you can whip up in a jiffy and enjoy with your whole family. You can even add more ingredients to make the dish healthier and more flavorful.

Time: 25 minutes

Serving Size: 2 servings

Prep Time: 5 minutes

Cook Time: 20 minutes

Ingredients for the scramble:

- ½ tsp avocado oil
- ½ tsp turmeric
- 1 cup of chickpeas (soaked overnight, boiled for an hour, drained, and dried; you can also use canned, but you must first rinse, drain, and dry)
- ¼ small onion (diced)
- 2 cloves of garlic (minced)
- Sea salt

Ingredients for the kale:

- ½ tsp avocado oil
- ½ tsp garlic (minced)
- 1 cup of kale leaves (stems removed, cut into small pieces)

Ingredients for assembling:

- ½ avocado (sliced)
- 2 small sweet potatoes (baked)

Directions:

1. In a pan, add the avocado oil over medium heat, along with the garlic and onions.
2. Cook for about 3 to 4 minutes until softened.
3. Add the chickpeas, turmeric, and salt, then continue cooking for about 10 more minutes. To avoid drying the mixture out, you may add teaspoons of water.
4. Mash about ⅔ of the chickpeas using a wooden spoon to make a scrambled texture.
5. Take the pan off the heat and set aside.
6. In a separate pan, add the avocado oil over medium heat, along with the garlic and kale.
7. Cook for about 5 minutes, until soft, then take the pan off the heat.
8. Slice one baked sweet potato in half and use a spoon to scoop out the center.
9. Spoon half of the chickpea scramble into the baked sweet potato and top with half of the softened kale.
10. Top with half of the avocado slices.
11. Repeat the assembling steps for the other baked sweet potato.
12. Serve immediately and enjoy.

High-Protein Breakfast Bowl

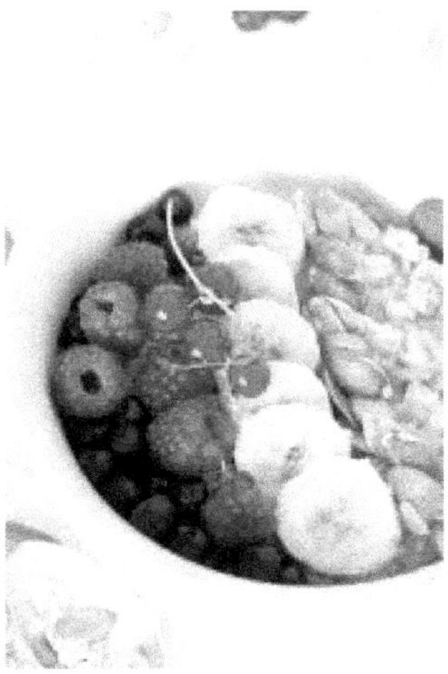

By enjoying a high-protein breakfast, you will have the energy to get you through the whole morning. This is a tasty and filling dish that you can also eat after a particularly intense workout. Apart from protein, this dish also contains healthy fats and complex carbs to give you all the nutrients you need to stay healthy while avoiding inflammation.

Time: 5 minutes

Serving Size: 1 serving

Prep Time: 5 minutes

Cook Time: no cooking time

Ingredients for the breakfast bowl:

- 1 ½ tbsp plant-based protein powder
- ¼ cup of blueberries
- ¼ cup of raspberries
- 1 small banana (sliced)
- 1 small sweet potato (baked)

Ingredients for the topping:

- Chia seeds

- Hemp hearts
- Other toppings of your choice

Directions:

1. Scoop out the flesh of the baked sweet potato and place it in a bowl.
2. Use a fork to mash the flesh until you get the consistency you desire.
3. Add the protein powder and mix until well combined.
4. Arrange the blueberries, raspberries, and banana slices in layers on top of the mashed sweet potato.
5. Top with your desired toppings.
6. Serve while warm or chill in the refrigerator for about 15 minutes before serving.

CHAPTER 4: LUNCH RECIPES FOR YOUR MEAL PLAN

Now that you have a bunch of amazing breakfast recipes, let's move on to the next meal of the day: lunch! By the time lunchtime rolls around, you've already used up almost all of your energy from your healthy anti-inflammatory breakfast. Your lunches can either be light or heavy, depending on what you have written on your meal plan. Of course, meal plans only serve as a guide. If you really want to succeed on the anti-inflammatory diet, try to practice some flexibility. As long as nothing on your plate promotes inflammation, you can enjoy and savor your meals to the very last bite!

Orange Chicken and Vegetables

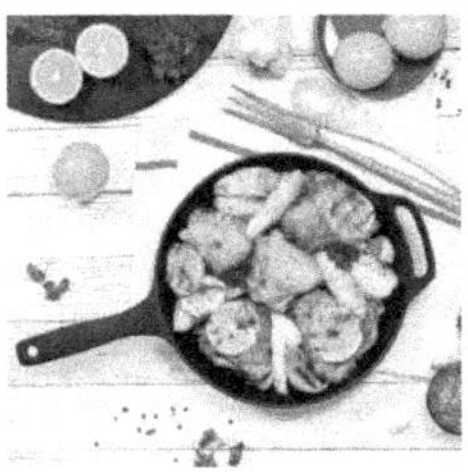

This super easy dish is perfect for lunch or dinner as it's savory, yummy, and filled with anti-inflammatory goodness. You will be cooking the juicy cuts of chicken with the veggies for a satisfying dish. And as a bonus, cleanup is a breeze because everything will be cooked in a single pan!

Time: 30 minutes

Serving Size: 2 servings

Prep Time: 5 minutes

Cook Time: 25 minutes

Ingredients:

- ¼ tsp black pepper (divided)
- ¼ tsp salt (divided)

- ½ tbsp tarragon (fresh, chopped)
- 1 ½ tbsp extra-virgin olive oil (divided)
- ¼ cup of chicken broth (low-sodium)
- 2 cups of sweet potatoes (slice each thin)
- 3 cups of baby kale
- ½ lb of chicken thighs (boneless, skinless, trimmed)
- 1 orange (sliced, seeded)
- 2 cloves of garlic (minced)

Directions:

1. Preheat your oven to 400°F.
2. In an oven-safe skillet, add ¾ tablespoon of the olive oil over medium-high heat.
3. Season each of the chicken thighs with salt and pepper and add to the skillet.
4. Cook each side for about 2 ½ minutes until browned, then transfer the chicken thighs to a plate.
5. Add the rest of the olive oil to the skillet along with the potatoes, with the cut side facing down, then sprinkle with salt and pepper.
6. Cook for about 3 minutes until browned.
7. Add the orange, garlic, tarragon, and chicken broth. Also, add the cooked chicken to the skillet.
8. Place the skillet in the oven and cook for about 15 minutes, until the potatoes are tender and the chicken is completely cooked through.
9. Take the skillet out of the oven, add the kale, then place it back in the oven.
10. Continue cooking for about 3 to 4 minutes, more until the kale has wilted.
11. Once cooked, take the skillet out of the oven and serve!

Oven-Baked Tilapia

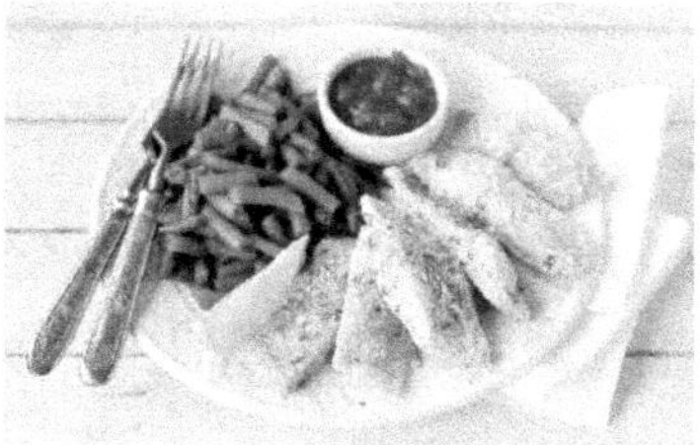

As you have already learned, fish is a fantastic source of protein and other essential nutrients to keep your body healthy. This recipe is easy, healthy, and oh-so-yummy! It includes the perfect blend of flavors and textures to give you a tasty lunch dish to enjoy with a refreshing glass of your favorite anti-inflammatory beverage.

Time: 30 minutes

Serving Size: 2 servings

Prep Time: 12 minutes

Cook Time: 18 minutes

Ingredients:

- ¼ tsp coconut palm sugar
- ¾ tsp olive oil
- 1 tsp rosemary (fresh, chopped)
- ¼ cup of breadcrumbs (whole-wheat)
- ¼ cup of pecans (raw, chopped)
- 1 egg (white only, you can also use store-bought egg replacers)
- 1 tilapia fillets
- Black pepper
- Cooking spray
- Salt

Directions:

1. Preheat your oven to 350°F.
2. In the baking dish, add the pecans, rosemary, sugar, breadcrumbs, olive oil, salt, and pepper, then toss everything together.
3. Place the baking dish in the oven and bake the pecan mixture for about 7 to 8 minutes.
4. Take the baking dish out of the oven and increase the heat to 400°F.
5. Use cooking spray to grease a larger baking dish.
6. In a dish, add the egg white and whisk.
7. Dip the tilapia fillets into the egg white, coat with the pecan mixture, and place in the baking dish.
8. If you have any remaining pecan mixture, sprinkle it on top of the tilapia fillets.
9. Place the baking dish in the oven and bake the tilapia fillets for about 10 minutes until just cooked through.
10. Take the baking dish out of the oven and serve with a side of steamed veggies or a cup of cooked quinoa.

Beef and Veggie Skillet

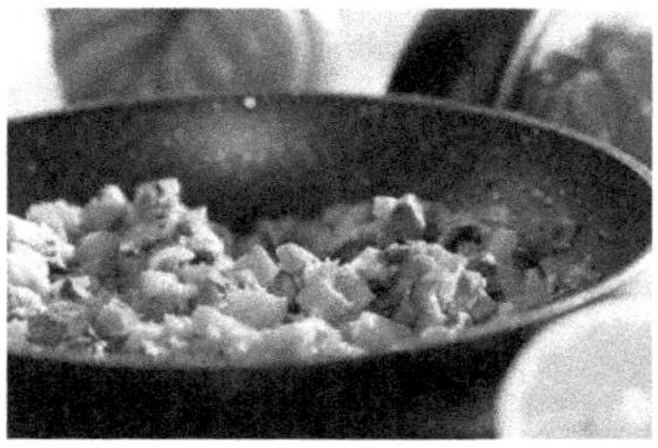

Beef and veggies go so well together that you can use this combination in different ways. For this recipe, you will be using lean, grass-fed beef along with different veggies to give you a nutrient-dense meal. This type of beef is healthier and, more importantly, it fits into your anti-inflammatory diet. Although red meat isn't one of the recommended food options on this diet, knowing which type of meat to choose for your recipes will allow you to enjoy red meat once in a while. This is another simple and quick meal that you can whip up for yourself no matter how busy your day gets.

Time: 20 minutes

Serving Size: 2 servings

Prep Time: 5 minutes

Cook Time: 15 minutes

Ingredients:

- 1 tsp sea salt
- 2 tsp ginger (ground)
- 1 tbsp avocado oil (you can also use olive oil)
- 1 lb ground beef (lean, grass-fed)
- 1 crown broccoli (chopped)
- 1 yellow squash (chopped)
- 2 carrots (peeled, chopped)
- 2 zucchini squash (chopped)
- 6 radishes (chopped)

Directions:

1. In a skillet, warm the avocado oil over medium heat.
2. Add the broccoli, carrots, and radishes, then stir well.
3. Cover the skillet with a lid and cook for about 5 minutes until the veggies have softened. Stir occasionally while cooking.
4. Remove the lid and move the veggies to one side.
5. Add the ground beef and create a flat layer.
6. Season with salt and ginger then cook for about 2 minutes until browned.
7. Flip the ground beef layer over then cook for about 2 minutes more.
8. Break the ground beef up and combine with the cooked veggies.
9. Add the yellow squash and zucchini squash to the mixture then cover.
10. Cook for about 5 minutes more until the ground beef is completely cooked through. Stir occasionally while cooking.
11. Once cooked, spoon into serving bowls and enjoy!

Charred Shrimp Buddha Bowl

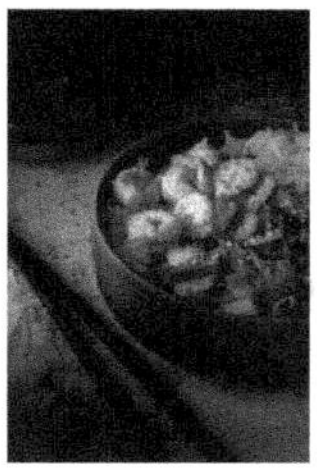

These Buddha bowls are so interesting that you can make them for your whole family for something healthy and delicious. Did you know the term "Buddha Bowl" comes from the fact that the dish has just the right balance? Since balance is one of the most important concepts in Buddhism, this title is just perfect! A wonderful thing about this recipe is that you can mix and match to suit your own tastes. For instance, you can add other yummy ingredients that will help calm the inflammation in your body each time you prepare this.

Time: 20 minutes

Serving Size: 2 servings

Prep Time: 15 minutes

Cook Time: 5 minutes

Ingredients:

- ½ tbsp extra-virgin olive oil
- 1 tbsp balsamic vinegar
- ¼ cup of pesto (homemade or store-bought)
- 1 cup of quinoa (cooked)
- 2 cups of arugula
- ½ lb large shrimp (peeled, deveined, patted dry)
- ½ avocado (diced)
- Black pepper
- Salt

- ½ cup of cherry tomatoes (optional, halved, you can also use olives instead)

Directions:

1. In a bowl, add the olive oil, vinegar, pesto, salt, and pepper, then whisk well.
2. Separate 2 tablespoons of the pesto mixture and set aside.
3. In a skillet, add the shrimp over medium-high heat. Cook for about 4 to 5 minutes until just cooked through and slightly charred.
4. Once cooked, transfer the shrimps to a plate.
5. In a bowl, add the quinoa, arugula, and the pesto mixture.
6. Toss lightly to coat.
7. Scoop the mixture into 2 bowls and top with avocado, tomatoes, and charred shrimp.
8. Drizzle with the remaining pesto mixture and serve!

Silky Avocado Pesto

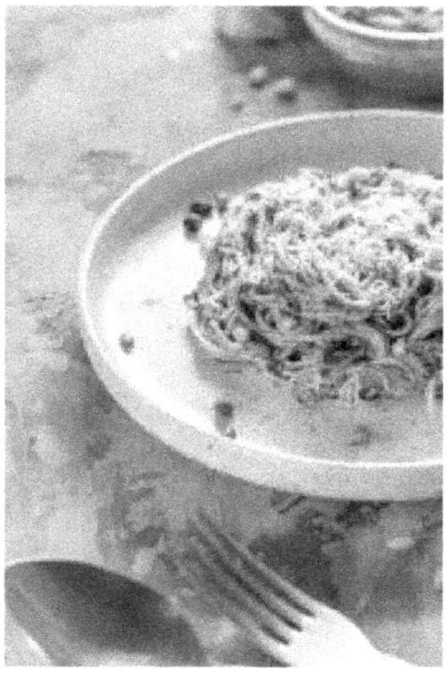

Pesto is a wonderful sauce for the anti-inflammatory diet as it is made of anti-inflammatory ingredients. This recipe makes pesto even healthier with the addition of avocado. Here, you will use the sauce for pasta, but you can also use it for other dishes like sandwiches or even salads. Once you know how to make the sauce, you can get creative with it!

Time: 15 minutes

Serving Size: 2 servings

Prep Time: 10 minutes

Cook Time: 5 minutes

Ingredients:

- 1 tbsp lemon juice
- ¼ cup of extra-virgin olive oil
- ¼ cup of pine nuts (you can also use walnuts)
- 1 bunch of basil (fresh)
- 2 avocados (ripe)
- 2 cloves of garlic
- Black pepper

- Sea salt
- 2 servings of pasta of your choice (cooked)

Directions:

1. Cook the pasta according to the package instructions. Once the pasta is cooked, drain the water, and set aside.
2. In a food processor, add the avocados, garlic, basil (leaves only), pine nuts, salt, and pepper, then pulse until all of the ingredients are finely chopped.
3. Add the oil and continue processing until you get a creamy and thick paste.
4. Add the pesto sauce to the pasta and toss to coat.
5. Serve while warm with a side of whole wheat garlic bread.

Poke Salad With Seared Tuna

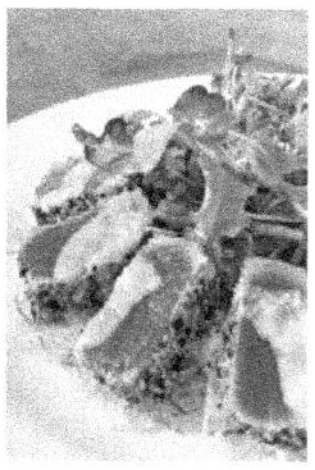

Salads are refreshing, healthy, and perfect for a light lunch. This salad is unique as it is topped with freshly-seared tuna. All of the flavors and textures in this dish add to its appeal, making it another winning addition to your diet. It's full of nutritious ingredients to make you happy and satisfied for the rest of the day—and it's super easy to make, too!

Time: 30 minutes

Serving Size: 2 servings

Prep Time: 15 minutes

Cook Time: 15 minutes

Ingredients for the tuna:

- ½ tsp cornstarch
- ½ tsp Sriracha
- 1 tbsp sesame seeds (black and white, toasted)
- ⅛ cup of honey
- ⅛ cup of pineapple juice
- ⅛ cup of soy sauce
- 1 ahi tuna steak
- 10 pieces of square-shaped wonton wrappers (cut into strips, you can also use corn tortillas)
- Cooking spray

Ingredients for the salad:

- ¼ cup of cilantro (fresh)

- ½ cup of pineapple (fresh, diced)
- 2 cups of spring greens (you can use any greens of your choice)
- ½ avocado (sliced)
- ½ jalapeño (sliced)

Ingredients for the dressing:

- ½ tsp sesame seeds (back and white, toasted)
- ½ tsp Sriracha
- 1 tsp ginger (fresh, grated)
- ½ tbsp tahini
- 1 tbsp pineapple juice
- 1 tbsp rice vinegar
- ⅛ cup of soy sauce
- ¼ cup of toasted sesame oil
- ½ lime (zest and juice)
- ½ clove of garlic (minced)

Directions:

1. Preheat your oven to 400°F and use cooking spray to grease a baking sheet.
2. Arrange the wonton strips on the baking sheet, grease with cooking spray, and season with sea salt.
3. Place the baking sheet in the oven and bake the wonton strips for about 5 to 10 minutes until they are crisp and have a light golden color.
4. Take the baking sheet out of the oven and set the wonton strips aside.
5. In a saucepot, add the soy sauce and cornstarch over medium heat and mix until you get a smooth texture.
6. Add the honey, pineapple juice, and Sriracha, mix well, and bring to a boil.

7. Once boiling, turn the heat down to low and allow to simmer for about 3 to 4 minutes until the sauce starts thickening. Remove from the heat and set aside.

8. In a skillet, add the sesame oil over high heat.

9. Once hot, place the tuna steak in the skillet and sear both sides for about 1 to 2 minutes each.

10. After searing the tuna steak, coat it with the soy sauce mixture.

11. Take the tuna steak out of the pan and slice it into strips.

12. In a bowl, add the salad ingredients and toss to mix.

13. In a separate bowl, mix together the dressing ingredients.

14. Spoon the salad onto plates and top with the wonton crisps and seared tuna.

15. Drizzle with dressing and serve immediately.

Skillet-Cooked Salmon

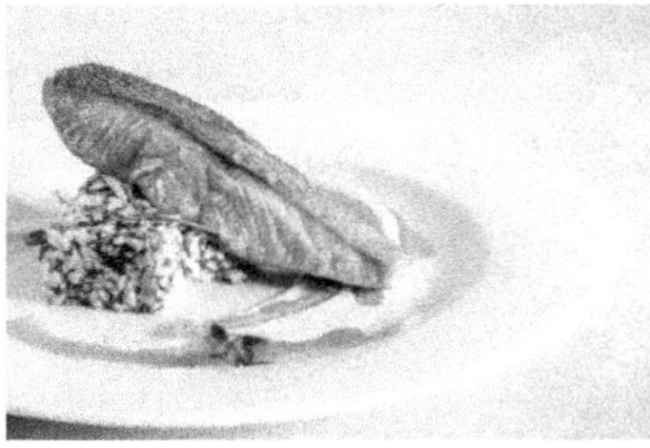

This salmon recipe will give you a lovely, crisp fillet with a flavorful and fresh sauce. You can serve it for lunch or dinner depending on what you're craving. This is another dish that's chock-full of anti-inflammatory goodness that fits right into your healthy meal plan. And if you want to share it with your family, all you have to do is double the quantities of the ingredients.

Time: 30 minutes

Serving Size: 2 servings

Prep Time: 10 minutes

Cook Time: 20 minutes

Ingredients for the salmon:

- ½ tsp paprika
- 1 tsp dill (dried)
- 1 tbsp avocado oil
- 1 lb salmon (cut into fillets)
- Sea salt

Ingredients for the sauce:

- 1 tsp dill (dried)
- 1 tsp lemon zest
- 1 tbsp lemon juice
- 1 ½ tbsp capers
- ½ cup of coconut milk

Directions:

1. Pat the salmon fillets dry using a paper towel, then season with dill, paprika, and sea salt.
2. In a skillet, warm the avocado oil over medium-high heat.
3. Once the oil is hot, add the salmon fillets with the flesh side facing down. Press the salmon fillets down lightly to ensure the whole surface is cooked.
4. Sear the salmon fillets for about 3 to 4 minutes until golden and crispy.
5. Flip the fillets and sear the skin side for about 2 to 3 minutes.
6. Flip the salmon once more and continue cooking for another 1 to 2 minutes.
7. Add the sauce ingredients to the skillet and whisk to combine, trying not to disturb the salmon fillets.
8. Continue cooking until the sauce thickens and the salmon fillets reach your desired level of doneness.
9. Spoon the salmon fillets and sauce onto plates and serve with cooked quinoa or steamed veggies for a hearty meal.

Greek-Style Turkey Burger

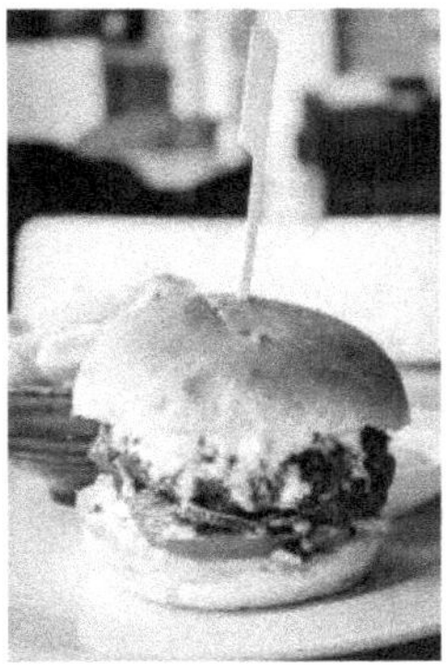

Have you ever tried turkey burgers before? If you haven't, this recipe will surely encourage you to be more adventurous with new types of food. This burger is served with an amazing tzatziki sauce that's flavorful and healthy. Since this burger uses turkey meat, it's lighter than traditional beef burgers, making it an excellent choice for dinner. Although this dish takes more than 30 minutes to make, the extra time will be worth it!

Time: 40 minutes

Serving Size: 2 servings

Prep Time: 10 minutes

Cook Time: 30 minutes

Ingredients for the burgers:

- ⅛ tsp red pepper flakes
- ¼ tsp oregano (dried)
- ½ tbsp extra virgin olive oil
- ¼ cup of parsley (fresh, chopped)
- ⅓ cup of bread crumbs
- ½ lb ground turkey
- ¼ red onion (sliced)
- ½ sweet onion (minced)

- 1 clove of garlic (minced)
- 1 egg (you can also use ⅓ cup of tofu or store-bought egg replacers)
- 2 hamburger buns (whole-wheat)
- 4 leaves of Boston lettuce
- Black pepper
- Cooking spray
- Salt
- 1 tomato (optional)

Ingredients for the sauce:

- ⅛ tsp garlic powder
- ½ tbsp extra-virgin olive oil
- 1 tbsp lemon juice (freshly squeezed)
- ⅛ cup of parsley (fresh, chopped)
- ½ cup of Greek yogurt
- ¼ European cucumber (diced)
- Black pepper
- Salt

Directions:

1. In a skillet, add the olive oil over medium heat, along with the onions.
2. Cook the onions for about 3 to 4 minutes until tender.
3. Add the garlic and continue cooking for about 1 minute until fragrant.
4. Take the skillet off the heat and allow to cool.
5. In a bowl, add the onion mixture along with the ground turkey, oregano, parsley, red pepper flakes, bread crumbs, salt, and pepper, then mix until well-combined.
6. Divide the mixture in half and form 2 turkey patties.
7. Preheat your oven to 375°F.

8. Grease an oven-safe skillet with cooking spray and warm over medium-high heat.

9. Add the turkey patties and brown each side for about 4 to 5 minutes each.

10. Place the skillet in the oven and continue cooking the turkey patties for about 13 to 15 minutes more.

11. While the patties are baking, make the sauce.

12. In a bowl, add the Greek yogurt, olive oil, lemon juice, garlic powder, cucumber, salt, and pepper, then mix until well-combined.

13. Gently stir the parsley into the sauce.

14. When the patties are done, take the skillet out of the oven and start assembling the burgers.

15. Place a turkey patty on the bottom bun, spread with the sauce, then top with tomato slices, lettuce leaves, and the top bun.

16. Serve immediately.

Anti-Inflammatory Green Curry

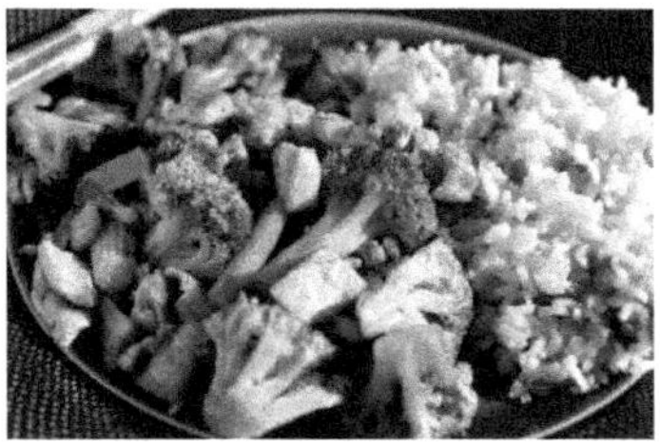

If you're looking for a recipe that's chock-full of vegetables, this is the one for you. It's easy to make your diet more interesting by learning to cook dishes that incorporate exotic flavors. This is one such dish, and when you get a taste of it, you will surely yearn for more. If you want, you can add more greens and veggies to this dish to make it even more satisfying and healthy.

Time: 30 minutes

Serving Size: 4 servings

Prep Time: 5 minutes

Cook Time: 25 minutes

Ingredients:

- ¼ tsp brown sugar
- ¼ tsp fish sauce
- 1 tbsp olive oil
- 2 tbsp green curry paste
- ¼ cup of golden raisins
- ½ cup of cilantro (fresh, chopped)
- ¾ cup of firm tofu
- 1 ½ cups of broccoli florets
- 2 ½ cups of coconut milk
- 1 sweet potato (peeled, cubed)
- Salt

Directions:

1. Remove excess water from the tofu by patting it dry with a paper towel, then cut the tofu into cubes.
2. In a soup pot, warm the olive oil over medium-high heat.
3. Add the tofu, season with salt, and fry for about 10 to 15 minutes.
4. Transfer the fried tofu cubes into a plate lined with a paper towel and set aside.
5. Add the coconut milk, curry paste, and sweet potatoes to the soup pot, and bring to a simmer. Continue simmering for about 5 minutes, until the sweet potatoes have become fork-tender.
6. Add the tofu and broccoli and continue simmering for about 5 minutes more.
7. As a final touch, add the fish sauce, brown sugar, cilantro, and golden raisins, then mix well.
8. Transfer the green curry into a serving bowl and serve hot with steamed brown rice.

Citrus Salad with Roasted Beets

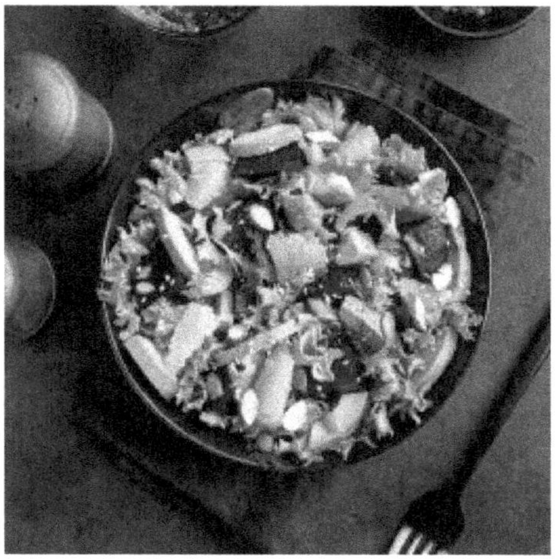

This salad is fresh, vibrant, and filled with wonderful flavors and textures. It's also packed with vitamins, minerals, and anti-inflammatory ingredients that will leave you feeling satisfied and energized. Although this dish might seem like a lighter option, it's actually quite filling thanks to the roasted beets.

Time: 15 minutes

Serving Size: 2 servings

Prep Time: 15 minutes

Cook Time: no cooking time

Ingredients for the salad:

- 1 tbsp hemp hearts (hulled)
- ¼ cup of baby arugula
- ¼ cup of baby spinach
- ¼ cup of pistachios (shelled)
- ½ avocado (peeled, cored, chopped)
- 1 small beet (roasted, cooled)
- 1 small blood orange (peeled, sectioned)
- 1 small clementine (peeled, sectioned)

Ingredients for the dressing:

- ¼ tsp oregano (dried)
- 1 ½ tbsp lemon juice (freshly squeezed)
- ⅛ cup of avocado oil (you can also use olive oil)
- Sea salt

Directions:

1. In a blender, add all of the dressing ingredients and blend until you get a smooth texture.
2. Add all of the salad ingredients to a bowl along with your desired amount of dressing. Toss until all of the salad ingredients are well coated.
3. Serve immediately and enjoy.

CHAPTER 5: DINNER RECIPES FOR YOUR MEAL PLAN

Your final meal of the day is very important, as it can spell the difference between a good night's sleep and a restless one. For instance, if you eat something that's too spicy for dinner, you might end up tossing and turning all night. But if you eat something healthy, satisfying, and not too heavy, you won't have to worry about waking up in the middle of the night because your tummy is bothering you. In this chapter, you will learn the final recipes you need for your meal plan. Before finalizing your meal plan, you can mix and match the dishes, then follow the recipes according to the sequence you have chosen.

Low-Carb Rice Bowl

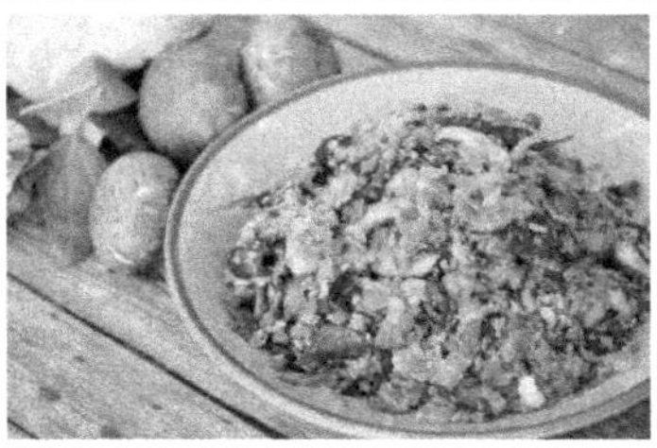

This low-carb dish is light enough for dinner and filling enough for lunch. It's low-carb because it includes "rice" that is actually made from cabbage instead of grains. It's clean, simple, and filled with healthy ingredients. Just like the other recipes presented here, you can also customize this according to your tastes. After you get the hang of making these simple dishes, you can start making versions with your own twist!

Time: 30 minutes

Serving Size: 1 to 2 servings

Prep Time: 5 minutes

Cook Time: 25 minutes

Ingredients for the turkey:

- 1 tsp ginger (ground)
- 1 tsp oregano (dried)
- 1 tsp sea salt
- 1 tbsp avocado oil

- 1 cup of mushrooms (chopped)
- 2 cups of baby spinach
- ½ lb ground turkey
- ½ apple (peeled, cored, sliced)
- ½ small yellow onion (diced)
- 1 zucchini squash (chopped)
- 3 cloves of garlic (minced)

Ingredients for the cabbage rice:

- ½ tsp sea salt
- 2 tbsp avocado oil
- 1 small head of green cabbage (grated)

Directions:

1. Add the cabbage into a food processor and pulse until you get cabbage bits the size of rice grains.
2. In a skillet, add the avocado oil over medium-high heat along with the cabbage rice and salt.
3. Cover the skillet and cook the cabbage rice for about 8 minutes, making sure that you stir frequently.
4. Once cooked, take the skillet off the heat and set aside.
5. In a separate skillet, add the avocado oil over medium-high heat, along with the apple and onion.
6. Cook for about 5 minutes until the onion starts turning translucent.
7. Add the mushrooms and continue cooking for 3 minutes more.
8. Move the veggies to one side, then add the ground turkey in a single layer.
9. Brown the ground turkey for 1 to 2 minutes, flip it over, and continue cooking for 1 to 2 minutes more.
10. Stir all of the ingredients in the skillet together.
11. Add the rest of the turkey ingredients then mix until well incorporated.
12. Cover the skillet with a lid and continue cooking for 5 minutes.
13. Spoon the cabbage rice into bowls and top with the turkey mixture.
14. Serve while hot.

Chicken and Veggie Stir-Fry

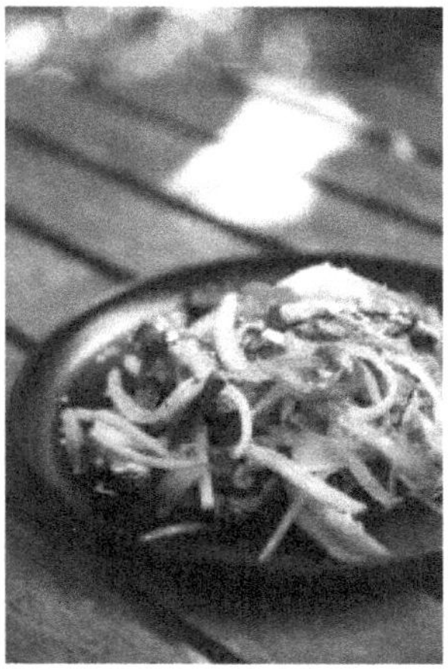

If you're not in the mood to cook but you really want to stick with your diet, here's an easy recipe for you. All you need are a couple of pantry staples to make this dish, plus a couple of minutes of stir-frying. It's tasty, simple, and much healthier than any stir-fry meals you will get from restaurants. Again, this is another recipe you can tweak to mix it up and include your favorite ingredients.

Time: 20 minutes

Serving Size: 2 servings

Prep Time: 10 minutes

Cook Time: 10 minutes

Ingredients:

- 1 tbsp rice vinegar
- 1 tbsp sesame seeds
- 1 tbsp olive oil
- 1 ½ tbsp cilantro (fresh, chopped)
- 1 ½ tbsp soy sauce (you can also use tamari)
- 1 ¼ cups of snap peas
- ¼ lb chicken breast (boneless, skinless, thinly sliced)
- ½ bunch of scallions (thinly sliced)

- ½ red bell pepper (thinly sliced)
- 1 clove of garlic (minced)
- Black pepper
- Salt
- 1 tsp Sriracha (optional)

Directions:

1. In a sauté pan, warm the olive oil over medium heat.
2. Add the garlic and scallions and sauté for about 1 minute until fragrant.
3. Add the snap peas and bell pepper, then continue sautéing for about 2 to 3 minutes more until just tender.
4. Add the chicken and cook for about 4 to 5 minutes until the veggies are tender and the chicken is fully cooked.
5. Add the rice vinegar, soy sauce, sesame seeds, and Sriracha if desired.
6. Toss all of the ingredients well to combine, then allow to simmer for about 1 to 2 minutes.
7. Spoon the stir-fry into bowls or plates and top with cilantro. Serve while hot.

Hearty Detox Salad

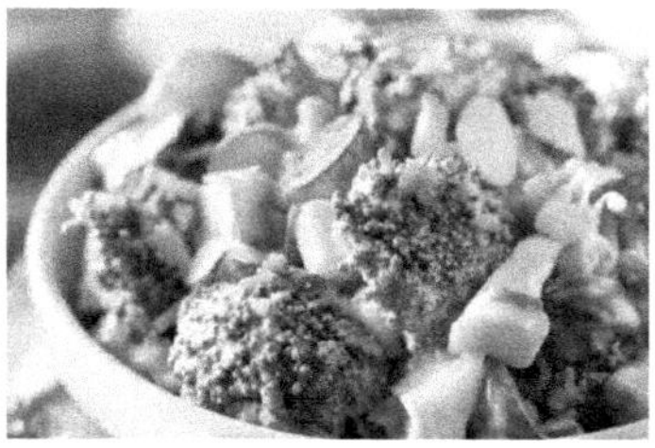

This is a nutritious salad that will help detox your body while reducing inflammation, too. It takes very little time and effort to make, but you will definitely feel the positive effects for a long time. Salads should always be part of your anti-inflammatory diet, especially if you're always on the go but you want to focus on eating healthy foods.

Time: 20 minutes

Serving Size: 2 servings

Prep Time: 15 minutes

Cook Time: 5 minutes

Ingredients for the salad:

- ½ cup of almonds (raw)
- 2 cups of baby kale
- 2 cups of broccoli florets (finely chopped)
- 2 cups of red cabbage (thinly sliced)
- ½ red bell pepper (thinly sliced)
- 1 large avocado (diced)
- 2 carrots (peeled, grated)
- 3 radishes (thinly sliced)
- 4 stalks of green onion (chopped)

Ingredients for the dressing:

- 2 tsp maple syrup

- 2 tsp stone-ground mustard
- ⅓ cup of avocado oil
- ⅓ cup of lemon juice (freshly squeezed)
- ½ cup of parsley (fresh)
- Sea salt

Directions:

1. In a blender, add all of the dressing ingredients and blend until everything is well-combined. Set aside.
2. Preheat your oven to 375°F.
3. Add the almonds to a baking sheet.
4. Place the baking sheet in the oven and roast the almonds for about 5 minutes.
5. Take the baking sheet out of the oven and allow the almonds to cool down before chopping.
6. In a bowl, add all of the salad ingredients.
7. Drizzle with the dressing and toss until all of the ingredients are well-coated.
8. Serve immediately with the remaining dressing on the side in case you want to add more to your salad.

** This recipe suggests that you add the broccoli florets raw to preserve their nutrient content. Just make sure to rinse thoroughly before chopping. You can also steam the broccoli florets lightly before adding them to the salad if desired.*

Pineapple-Sweetened Fried Rice

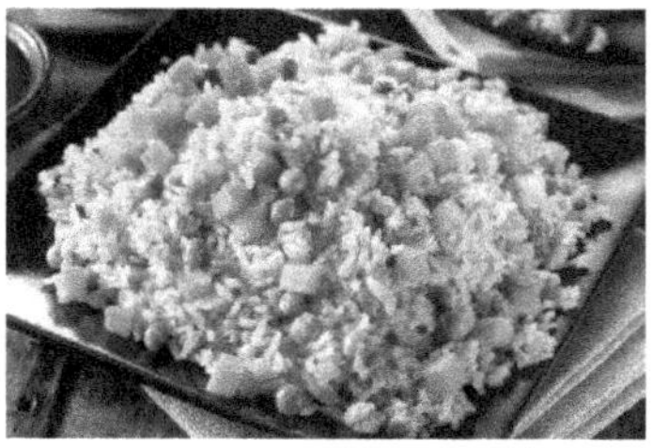

This is another quick, easy, and tasty meal that you can eat on its own or pair it with a light and healthy protein like steamed fish. Pineapple is one of the most anti-inflammatory fruits you can eat, and this dish is sweetened by this fruit. It has wonderful flavors and it's filling enough to make you feel satisfied, yet not so heavy to make you feel too full.

Time: 30 minutes

Serving Size: 2 servings

Prep Time: 10 minutes

Cook Time: 20 minutes

Ingredients:

- ¼ tsp ginger (powdered)
- ½ tbsp sesame oil
- 1 tbsp olive oil
- 1 ½ tbsp soy sauce
- ¼ cup of corn (frozen)
- ¼ cup of peas (frozen)
- 1 cup of pineapple (fresh or canned, diced)
- 1 ½ cups of brown rice (cooked)
- ½ onion (diced)
- 1 carrot (peeled, grated)
- 1 clove of garlic (minced)

- 1 green onion (sliced)
- White pepper

Directions:

1. In a bowl, add the sesame oil, ginger powder, soy sauce, and white pepper, then mix well. Set aside.
2. In a wok, add the olive oil over medium-high heat, along with the onion and garlic.
3. Cook for about 3 to 4 minutes until the onions start turning translucent.
4. Add the peas, corn, and carrots, then continue cooking for about 3 to 4 minutes more until the veggies are tender.
5. Add the pineapple, rice, green onions, and the sauce mixture.
6. Stir constantly for about 2 minutes until everything is completely heated through.
7. Serve while hot!

Mediterranean-Style Cod

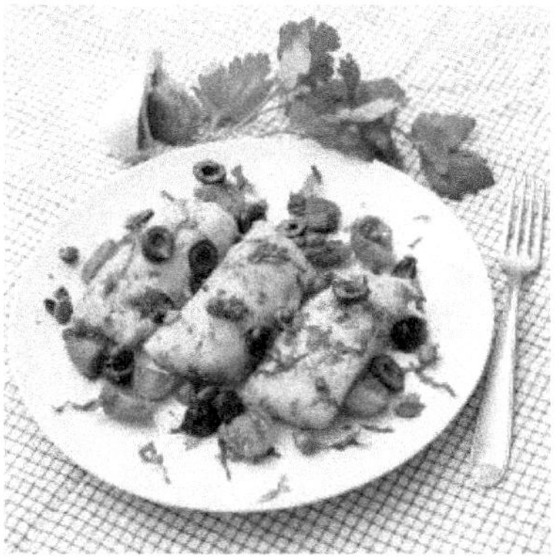

This Mediterranean-inspired dish takes only a few minutes to make, yet it offers amazingly complex flavors. It's colorful, flavorful, and nutrient-dense. You can use different types of white fish for this dish to get all the wonderful benefits various fish have to offer. Whether you whip this up for yourself or serve it at a party, you will surely enjoy every single bite.

Time: 15 minutes

Serving Size: 2 servings

Prep Time: 5 minutes

Cook Time: 10 minutes

Ingredients:

- ⅛ teaspoon garlic powder
- ⅛ teaspoon paprika
- 1 tsp capers
- 1 tsp oregano (fresh, snipped)
- 1 tsp thyme (fresh, snipped)
- ½ tbsp olive oil
- 1 tbsp ripe olives (pitted, sliced)
- ½ sprig of oregano (fresh, you can also use thyme)
- 1 clove of garlic (sliced)

- 2 cod fillets (frozen or fresh, skinless)
- Black pepper
- Cooking spray
- Salt
- 1 ½ cups of cherry tomatoes (optional, you can also use olives instead)

Directions:

1. Preheat your oven to 450°F.
2. Use foil to line a baking pan and grease it with cooking spray.
3. Use a paper towel to pat the fish fillets dry.
4. In a bowl, combine the thyme, oregano, paprika, garlic powder, salt, and pepper, then mix well.
5. Coat the fish fillets with the spice mixture generously and evenly.
6. Place the fillets on one side of the baking pan. On the other side, add the garlic and tomatoes.
7. Add oil to the rest of the spice mixture, whisk, and drizzle it over the veggies. Toss until well coated.
8. Place the baking pan in the oven and bake for about 8 to 12 minutes.
9. Add the capers and olives to the cooked veggies and mix well.
10. Transfer the fish and veggies onto plates and garnish with fresh oregano. Serve while hot.

Roasted Sheet-Pan Veggies

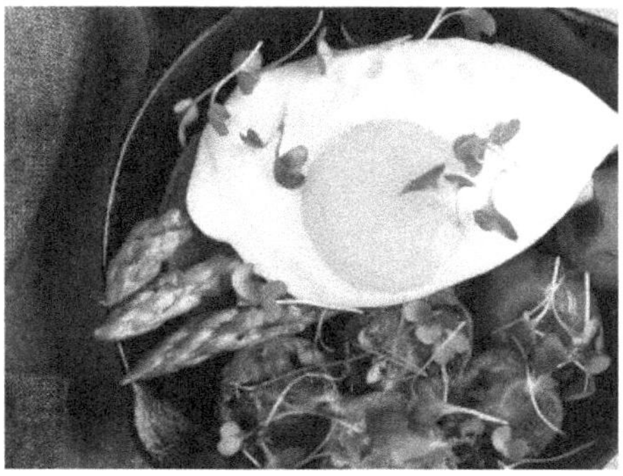

This easy recipe makes for a healthy meal that you can serve for dinner or at any time of the day. One of the main ingredients is eggs, but if you have noticed that your body doesn't react well to eggs, you can replace this ingredient. Since this dish also contains veggies, you're sure to have a nutrient-dense meal to make you satisfied.

Time: 30 minutes

Serving Size: 2 servings

Prep Time: 10 minutes

Cook Time: 20 minutes

Ingredients:

- 1 tsp thyme (fresh, chopped)
- 1 tbsp olive oil
- 1 cup of asparagus
- 2 eggs (you can also use ⅓ cup of cubed tofu or store-bought egg replacers)
- Black pepper
- Cooking spray
- Salt
- 1 cup of cherry tomatoes (optional, you can also use olives instead)

Directions:

1. Preheat your oven to 400°F and use cooking spray to grease a baking sheet.
2. Add the cherry tomatoes and asparagus to the baking sheet and spread them evenly in a single layer.
3. Drizzle olive oil over the veggies and season with salt, pepper, and thyme. Toss lightly to coat the veggies.
4. Place the baking sheet in the oven and roast the veggies for about 10 to 12 minutes.
5. Take the baking sheet out of the oven and crack the eggs on top of the veggies. Season the eggs with salt and pepper.
6. Place the baking sheet back in the oven and continue roasting for about 7 to 8 minutes more.
7. Once cooked, take the baking sheet out of the oven and divide the veggies evenly onto plates. Serve while hot!

Refreshing Salad with Crunchy Chickpeas

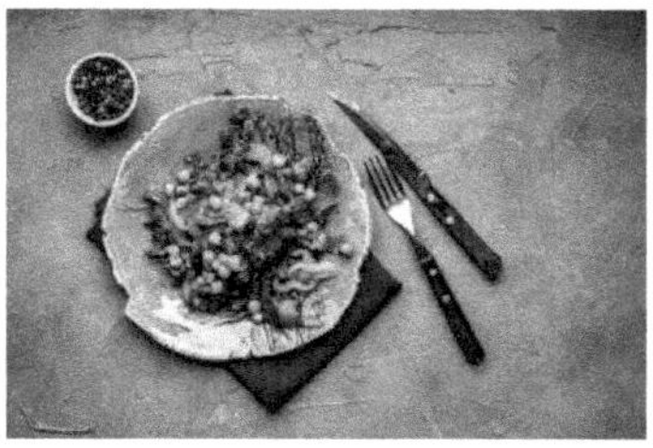

This salad is a bit more filling than what we're normally used to, but you can always get a smaller portion if you think it's too heavy. It has amazing Middle Eastern flavors along with crunchy chickpeas to add some texture. This meal is flavorful, filling, and completely plant-based! It even comes with a creamy sauce that's oh-so-delicious.

Time: 30 minutes

Serving Size: 2 servings

Prep Time: 10 minutes

Cook Time: 20 minutes

Ingredients for the chickpeas:

- ¼ tsp cardamom
- ¼ tsp coriander (ground)
- ¼ tsp ginger (ground)
- ½ tsp cinnamon (ground)
- ½ tsp smoked paprika
- ½ tsp turmeric
- 1 tsp cumin
- 1 tbsp olive oil
- 2 cups of chickpeas (soaked overnight, boiled for an hour, drained, and dried; you can also use canned, but you must first rinse, drain, and dry)
- Sea salt
- Black pepper

Ingredients for the salad:

- ¼ cup of red onion (thinly sliced)
- ½ cup of quinoa (cooked)
- ⅔ cup of spring mix lettuce (preferably organic)
- ¾ cup of parsley (fresh)
- 10 cherry tomatoes (optional, chopped, you can also use olives instead)

Ingredients for the dressing:

- 1 tsp dill (dried)
- 2 tbsp lemon juice (freshly squeezed)
- ½ cup of hummus (store-bought or homemade)
- 3 cloves of garlic (finely minced)
- Water (for thinning)

Directions:

1. Preheat your oven to 400°F and place a rack in the middle.
2. In a bowl, add all of the chickpea ingredients and toss until well combined.
3. Use a fork to mash half of the chickpeas.
4. Add the chickpeas to a baking sheet and place in the oven.
5. Bake the chickpeas for about 20 to 22 minutes.
6. While baking, add all of the salad ingredients, except for the quinoa, to a bowl. Toss to combine, then set aside.
7. In a separate bowl, add all of the ingredients except the water. Whisk well.
8. Add water to the dressing until you get a pourable texture.
9. When the chickpeas are done, take the baking sheet out of the oven and prepare the salad.
10. Add the quinoa to the salad and toss lightly.
11. Divide the salad into bowls or plates and drizzle with dressing.
12. Top with crunchy chickpeas and serve immediately.

Fresh and Healthy Shrimp Wrap

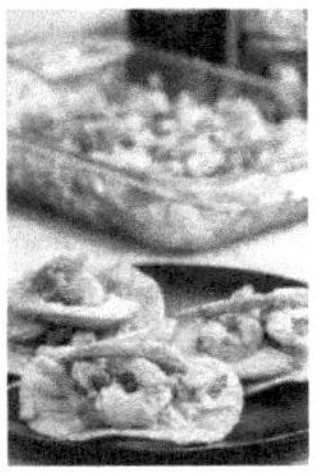

This is one of the quickest and easiest recipes you can prepare for yourself, making it perfect for your busiest day of the week. You can either buy cooked shrimp or you can buy shelled and deveined shrimp for easier cooking. These satisfying wraps are so tasty, you might want to make a bigger batch in case one isn't enough.

Time: 5 minutes

Serving Size: 1 serving

Prep Time: 5 minutes

Cook Time: no cooking time

Ingredients:

- 1 tbsp lime juice
- 2 tbsp feta cheese (crumbled)
- ¼ cup of avocado (diced)
- ¾ cup of shrimp (cooked, chopped)
- 1 scallion (sliced)
- 1 tortilla wrap (whole-wheat)
- ¼ cup of cherry tomatoes (optional, diced, you can also use olives instead)

Directions:

1. In a bowl, combine all of the ingredients except the tortilla wrap and toss well.
2. Scoop the mixture onto the tortilla wrap and fold it over nicely.
3. Serve immediately.

Quinoa Salad With Salmon

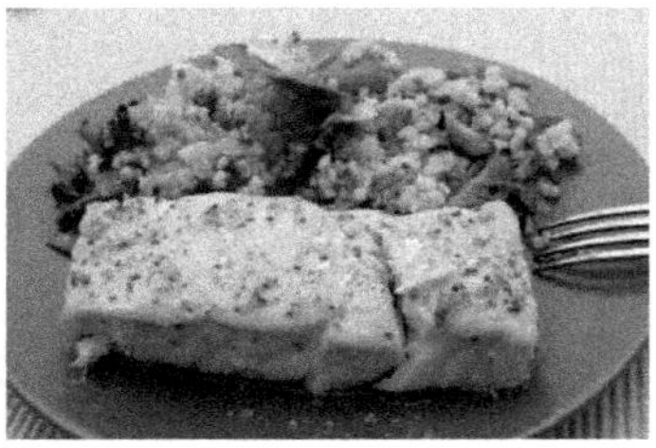

This salad has a unique zesty flavor combined with a Mediterranean flair. It features salmon, which is one of the healthiest fish on the planet. Just make sure to choose wild salmon, as this is much healthier and more anti-inflammatory compared to farm-raised fish. You can make this salad and eat it right away or store it in the refrigerator for later. Either way, this is an amazing dish to have for dinner.

Time: 15 minutes

Serving Size: 2 servings

Prep Time: 5 minutes

Cook Time: 10 minutes

Ingredients:

- ¼ tsp pepper (divided)
- ¼ tsp salt (divided)
- 1 tbsp red-wine vinegar
- 1 ½ tbsp extra-virgin olive oil (divided)
- ⅛ cup of cilantro (fresh, chopped)
- ⅛ cup of pistachios (toasted, chopped)
- ½ cup of red bell peppers (roasted, chopped)
- 1 cup of quinoa (cooked)
- ¾ lb salmon (preferably wild-caught, skin-on, cut in half)
- 1 clove of garlic (grated)

Directions:

1. In a skillet, warm ¾ tablespoon of olive oil over medium-high heat.
2. Use a paper towel to pat the salmon fillets dry, then season each fillet with half of the salt and pepper.
3. Add the salmon fillets to the skillet with the flesh side facing down and cook for about 3 to 4 minutes.
4. Flip the salmon fillets over and continue cooking for about 1 to 2 minutes more.
5. Once cooked, transfer the salmon fillets to plates.
6. In a bowl, add the vinegar, garlic, and the remaining olive oil, salt, and pepper.
7. Add the pistachios, cilantro, red peppers, and quinoa, then toss to combine.
8. Spoon the salad next to the salmon fillets on the plates and serve immediately.

Mediterranean Vegetable Wraps

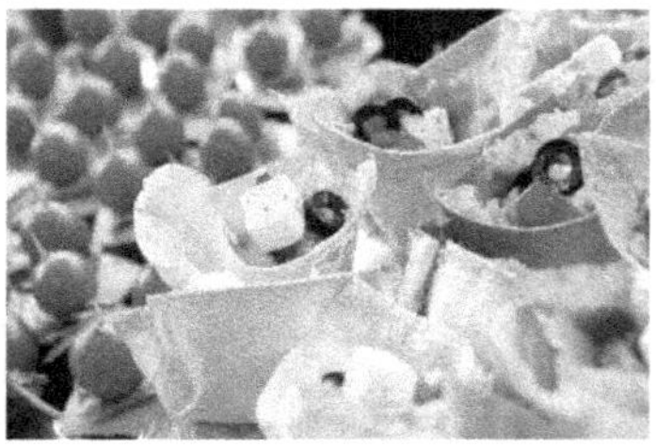

These nutritious wraps are filled with healthy veggies and other savory ingredients. You can prepare the hummus days before and store it in the refrigerator so that all you have to do is prepare the veggies and assemble the wraps. You can also make the hummus and enjoy it fresh with your veggie wraps.

Time: 15 minutes

Serving Size: 2 servings

Prep Time: 15 minutes

Cook Time: no cooking time

Ingredients for the hummus:

- ½ tbsp tahini
- 1 tbsp olive oil
- 1 ½ tbsp lemon juice (freshly squeezed)
- ⅛ cup of cilantro leaves (fresh)
- 1 cup of chickpeas (soaked overnight, boiled for an hour, drained, and dried; you can also use canned, but you must first rinse and drain)
- ½ clove of garlic (peeled)
- Salt
- White pepper

Ingredients for the wraps:

- ½ tbsp balsamic vinegar
- ½ tbsp olive oil

- ⅛ cup of feta cheese (crumbled)
- ¼ cup of red onion (thinly sliced)
- ½ cup of tomato (chopped)
- 2 cups of mixed baby greens
- ½ clove of garlic (minced)
- ½ small cucumber (sliced into strips)
- 2 multi-grain wraps
- Black pepper

Directions:

1. In a food processor, add all of the hummus ingredients then process until you get a smooth, thick, and creamy texture.
2. In a bowl, add the cucumber, red onion, tomato, mixed greens, and feta cheese. Toss to combine.
3. In a separate bowl, add the olive oil, black pepper, and garlic. Whisk well.
4. Drizzle the dressing over the salad and toss until well-combined.
5. Spread the whole-wheat wraps with hummus and top with the salad.
6. Wrap, then serve immediately.

CHAPTER 6: ANTI-INFLAMMATORY SNACK OPTIONS

With a well-made meal plan, you can motivate yourself to continue choosing anti-inflammatory foods all day, every day. Creating meal plans will also help you become more aware of inflammatory and anti-inflammatory foods. The more you practice (through meal planning), the more familiar you will become with the foods that fit into your diet. Apart from breakfast, lunch, and dinner, you will likely also eat snacks once in a while.

Snacks are a normal part of our day. If you want to avoid inflammation, you don't have to restrict yourself from eating snacks, especially if you feel hungry after meals. The key here is to know which snacks to eat and which to avoid. By choosing the right snacks, you can keep your body nourished throughout the day with healthy, nutritious food that will reduce or even prevent inflammation. In this chapter, we will explore the healthiest anti-inflammatory snacks to include in your diet.

The Best Snack Options

If you find yourself sitting at home or in the office and you realize that you're hungry, what should you do? For one, you shouldn't restrict yourself. Restricting yourself from eating something if you're hungry can cause you stress, especially if it happens all the time. Stress is another factor that may cause inflammation in your body, so you should avoid this, too. Snacking can be an enjoyable and satisfying experience as long as you choose healthy foods, such as:

Avocados

Avocados are super healthy and they can be used in different kinds of dishes. The best part is, you can also eat avocados on their own. Apart from containing healthy fats, avocados are chock-full of other nutrients and antioxidants, many of which have anti-inflammatory effects. Aside from eating avocados on their own, you can have them in sandwiches, salads, or even smoothies.

Blueberries

Blueberries are considered a superfood because of all the antioxidants they contain. These tiny berries are rich in polyphenols, which promote antioxidant production in the body. All of these healthy things protect your body against inflammation. Fortunately, blueberries are very easy to enjoy as a snack. All you have to do is grab a handful and start eating!

Broccoli

Broccoli is a great option for a snack. This veggie is rich in glucosinolates, a type of antioxidant that makes your body healthy and strong. It also contains a lot of fiber, making it a wonderful low-calorie snack option. Enjoy it steamed, baked with a little bit of salt, or even raw and crunchy!

Carrots

Carrot sticks are a very healthy and popular snack. This veggie contains a lot of antioxidants that will reduce your inflammation while increasing your overall health and wellness. Aside from eating your carrots raw, you can also pan-fry them or roast them for a wonderfully tasty snack.

Cauliflower popcorn

Here's another great snack option for you—simply toss a bunch of cauliflower florets in oil, season with some salt, and roast it in the oven for about 30 minutes. You can use different seasonings and spice blends to keep things interesting. Cauliflower is almost as healthy as broccoli and it also contains fiber. If you don't want to make popcorn (or you don't have time), then you can eat this veggie raw, too.

Dark chocolate

If you need something sweet to satisfy your sweet tooth, then a piece of dark chocolate is a perfect choice. When it comes to dark chocolate, opt for those made with at least 60% cacao to get the beneficial polyphenol content that helps reduce inflammation. Also, choose dark chocolate that doesn't contain a lot of added sugar since sugar tends to promote inflammation.

Guacamole

Since guacamole is made from avocados, it's definitely a healthy option. You can make guacamole right in your own kitchen—it's super easy to make. Then you can enjoy your guacamole with whole-grain tortilla chips or even fresh vegetable sticks. This snack is perfectly filling, healthy, and anti-inflammatory.

Hard-boiled eggs

If you already know that eggs don't affect you negatively, then you can enjoy them as a healthy snack. The easiest way to enjoy eggs is by hard-boiling them and eating them as is. It's best to hard boil a batch of eggs so that you always have a ready-to-eat snack whenever you feel hungry. Of course, you can also cook healthy egg-based snacks, but these may take more time and effort.

Hummus

Just like guacamole, hummus is a wonderful snack dip made from healthy ingredients. This time, you will use chickpeas as the main ingredient to make your own creamy hummus to pair with baby carrots, veggie sticks, sugar snap peas, or whole-wheat tortilla chips. Hummus also adds more protein and fiber to your diet to keep you healthy and strong.

Kale chips

If you love kale in your salads, then you will love it as baked chips, too. Kale contains iron, potassium, vitamins, and other nutrients that reduce inflammation. Roast your own kale chips at home or buy organic store-bought kale chips. Make sure to read the label of the chips so that you can choose the healthiest option available.

Kombucha

If you love soda, you will be happy to know that kombucha can satisfy your soda cravings. Kombucha is a black tea beverage that has been fermented. It is cheap and refreshingly fizzy, but it doesn't come with all of the unhealthy ingredients that sodas are filled with. Instead, it contains live probiotics to improve the health of your gut and help your body in various ways. Your gut plays an important role in managing inflammation. This means that if you have a healthy gut, it will help your body keep inflammation at bay. While you can make kombucha at home, most people simply buy their beverages since they are affordable.

Oranges

Oranges contain folate, vitamins, and other nutrients that have anti-inflammatory effects. In particular, the vitamin C content of oranges helps protect you from illnesses while fighting off inflammation. If you feel yourself craving something refreshing and sweet, grab an orange and enjoy!

Roasted almonds (lightly salted)

Almonds are one of the healthiest nuts available and they make for a quick, convenient snack. These nuts contain fiber, magnesium, and omega-3s, all of which combat inflammation. Roasted almonds are probably the tastiest way to enjoy almonds, as long as you opt for lightly-salted varieties. Keep in mind, it's very easy to overindulge in almonds and other nuts so it's best to take a handful to snack on instead of eating the almonds straight from the bag or can.

Smoothies

Smoothies are very trendy these days because they are healthy, filling, and super easy to make. You can also make different types of smoothies simply by mixing and matching ingredients. The best types of smoothies are those which contain fresh fruits and veggies. You can even add anti-inflammatory spices like turmeric and ginger to boost the nutrient content of your smoothies. Perfect!

Sweet potato fries

Sweet potatoes help reduce inflammation in the body since they contain a lot of essential vitamins. Sweet potatoes contain beta-carotene, an extremely powerful antioxidant with anti-inflammatory properties. Instead of munching on French fries, make your own sweet potato fries at home. These are just as good but they contain more vitamins and minerals that will benefit your health.

Toasted chickpeas

This is another amazing savory and crunchy treat to make from home. Instead of opening bags of chips that are full of preservatives, salt, and oil, make your own batch of roasted chickpeas from home. Simply season the chickpeas with olive oil and your own mix of spices and roast them in the oven. Chickpeas contain complex carbs, making them a much better choice than processed savory snacks.

Trail mix

Trail mix is healthy, interesting, and completely customizable. Again, it's best to make your own trail mix instead of buying from supermarkets, as many of the trail mix products contain added salt or sugar, which won't help you prevent inflammation. Make your own trail mix by combining nuts, seeds, banana chips, dried goji berries, dried cranberries, and even dark chocolate chunks. You can add a bit of salt to the mix then store your homemade masterpiece in an airtight container for a convenient snacking option.

Zucchini chips

These chips are a great appetizer and a wonderful snack, too. You can coat zucchini slices with almond flour and either fry or bake them to make them crispy. Snacking on veggies will help you become healthier and when you make your own veggie chips, this will make it easier for you to get used to veggies. Soon, eating raw vegetables will become your new normal!

As you can see, snacking on anti-inflammatory foods doesn't have to be challenging because there are many options for you to choose from. There are even more complex snack recipes you can whip up on weekends when you have time to spare.

The Worst Snack Options

There will always be another side to any story. Just as there are healthy, anti-inflammatory snack options for you to munch on, there are also certain foods that you should avoid as much as possible, as they tend to promote or even cause inflammation. Some examples of such snacks are:

Buttery crackers

Although buttery crackers taste great, they don't even make you feel full. What's worse, they don't contain the nutrients your body needs to stay healthy. This means that essentially, they are empty calories. Most of these crackers are made with refined flour, added colors or flavors, and hydrogenated oils, all of which promote inflammation. Instead of these crackers, satisfy your cravings with something healthier like roasted chickpeas or whole-wheat tortilla chips with hummus dip.

Crunchy snacks with orange cheese-flavored powder

You have probably seen these snacks before because they are practically everywhere! From chips to cheese puffs and everything in between, orange-colored snacks are very popular. Unfortunately, that orange cheese-flavored powder causes irritation and inflammation in the body. Aside from this, such snacks typically contain trans fats, too, another inflammatory ingredient. If you're craving cheese, try feta or goat cheese. Or you can snack on the savory options presented in the previous section, which are healthier and more filling.

Microwave popcorn

Generally, popcorn is considered a healthy snack because it's low in calories but it contains good amounts of fiber. But products like microwave popcorn are a different story. Microwave popcorn typically contains added flavorings, chemicals, and hydrogenated fats, which tend to trigger inflammation. Although this type of popcorn is more convenient, you should put in the extra time and effort to make your own popcorn at home. Then you can season it using healthy ingredients to make a sweet or savory fiber-rich snack.

Specialty coffee

Snacking on a cold glass of coffee from cafés and coffee shops seems like a good idea, especially since you won't be "eating" anything. However, these specialty coffee drinks contain tons of sugar, which promotes inflammation. Although coffee has anti-inflammatory properties, if you drink it with milk, sugar, chocolate sauce, and whipped cream, all these other ingredients won't make this an ideal snack for you. If you want or need a caffeine fix, go for black coffee or tea instead.

Store-bought granola bars

Granola bars are considered healthy foods and because of this, many people buy granola bars when they're on a diet. However, most processed granola bars contain very little fiber, protein, and nutrients. Instead, they contain a lot of added sugar, making them a lot like candy bars. If you can make your own granola bars at home using anti-inflammatory ingredients, you can add this option to your anti-inflammatory snacks. Otherwise, it's best to find something healthier to satisfy your sweet tooth.

Whenever you want to purchase your snacks instead of making them from home, don't forget to check the labels. If you see any ingredients on the list that promotes inflammation, find something else. That way, you don't have to feel guilty or worried whenever you give in to your snack cravings.

CPSIA information can be obtained
at www.ICGtesting.com
Printed in the USA
LVHW051936060821
694730LV00005B/725

9 781802 448498